THE GIFT OF MOTHERHOOD

Your personal journey through prepared childbirth

Introduction

The birth of your baby is a life changing event and a moment that you will remember always. Your journey may be filled with excitement, joy and a slight fear of the unknown. The purpose of this information is to help you understand the process of labor and birth and to answer questions about the birth of your child. The more knowledge you have of the process of birth, the more likely you will approach your personal journey with confidence.

This information is for general reference purposes only and cannot be relied upon as a substitute for medical care. You should have regular prenatal checkups and also consult with your healthcare provider about any special health questions or concerns. Every person is unique and may require a special treatment program.

Special thanks to the many people all over the country who helped with suggestions, advice and support. Without their expertise and guidance, this publication could not have been produced in an accurate and complete way.

FREE DIGITAL ACCESS

This book includes a digital enhancement.
Access your book content, watch videos, log feedings and more — from any device, anywhere. Everytime you see in this book, log into YoMingo for access to corresponding content.

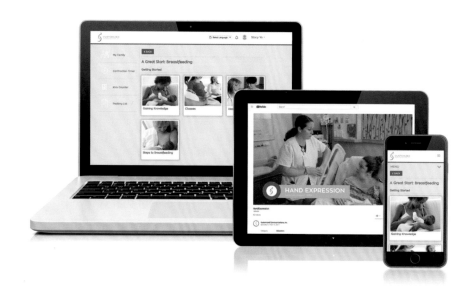

Simply scan this QR code for FREE access or visit:

customizedinc.com/TheGiftofMotherhood

Powered by **YOMINGO**

Table of Contents

Please Note: All words highlighted in *Blue* are clearly defined in the glossary.

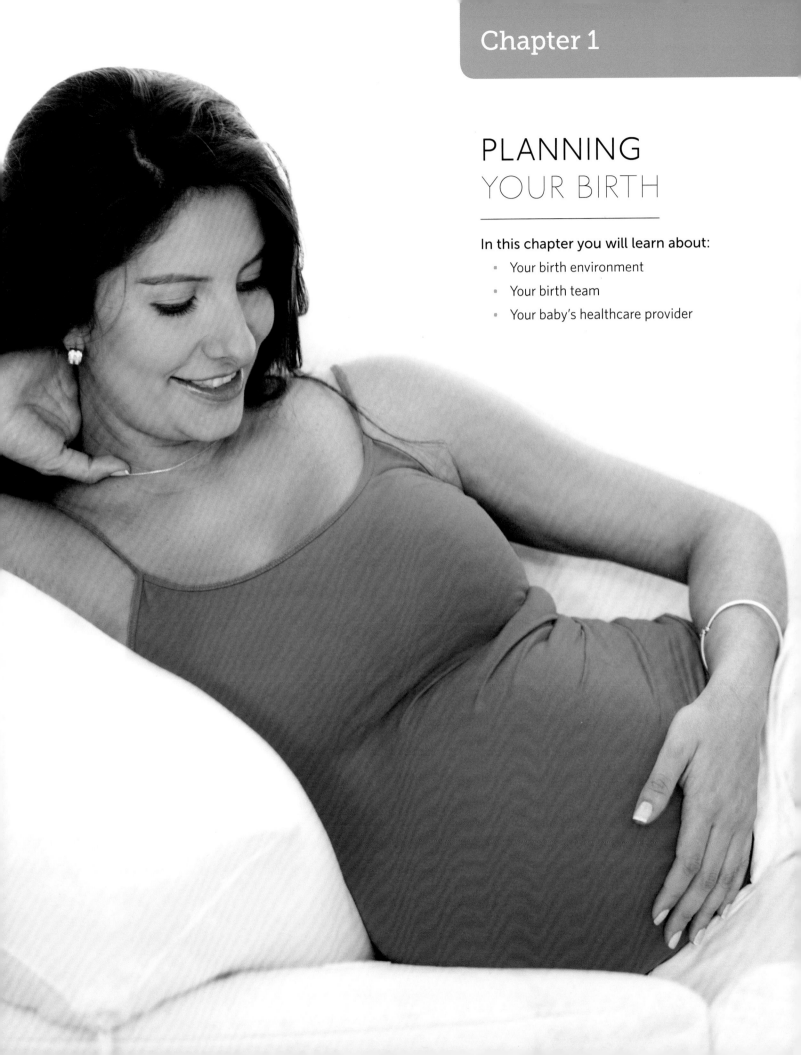

Chapter 1

PLANNING
YOUR BIRTH

In this chapter you will learn about:

- Your birth environment
- Your birth team
- Your baby's healthcare provider

Birth Environment

You need to consider where you are going to give birth early in your pregnancy. It is also important to communicate effectively with your physician or healthcare provider on the management of your labor and birth. Understanding the policies of the hospital or birthing center is especially important if you have a particular birth plan in mind. Ask yourself and your healthcare provider what choices will result in a birth experience with the best possible outcome.

Hospital Setting

Most hospitals have set days and times for tours. Hospitals have developed tours to provide information to families who are shopping for hospitals to educate expectant families about hospital services. The hospital or birthing center you choose will largely depend on your insurance carrier, healthcare provider and the services provided.

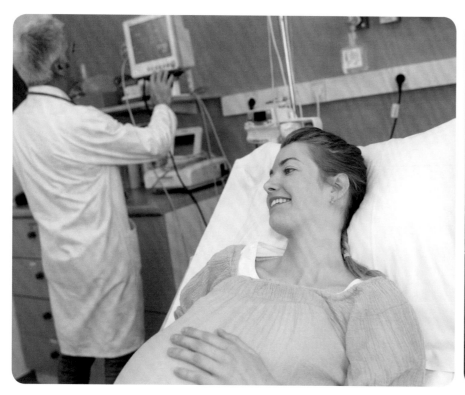 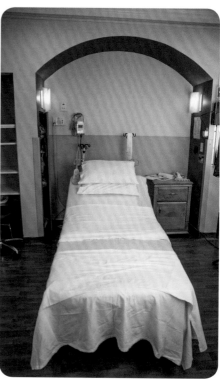

Things to consider when choosing a hospital:

- Does the facility offer birthing rooms?
- Are there LDR's (labor, delivery, recovery rooms) or LDRP's (labor, delivery, recovery and *postpartum* rooms)?
- What is the hospital's policy on rooming-in?
- Why would my baby have to go to the nursery?
- How many people are allowed in the room at the time of birth?
- What are the visiting hours?
- Are siblings allowed at any time or are there age restrictions on sibling visitation?
- Are there breastfeeding educators or lactation consultants on staff?
- What, if any, security does the facility have for taking special care of my newborn?
- If a *cesarean birth* is necessary, where will it be performed?
- Will my support person be allowed in the surgical room if I need a cesarean?

Birthing Center

Birthing centers have become very popular. These centers encourage natural childbirth. It is the philosophy of the centers that childbirth is a natural process that is not meant to be a technical or medical procedure. They are usually run by a nurse-midwife who has been certified and may or may not have a physician overseeing the facility. Just as in choosing a hospital, there are many things that you must also consider in choosing a birthing center.

Questions you need to ask your birthing center:

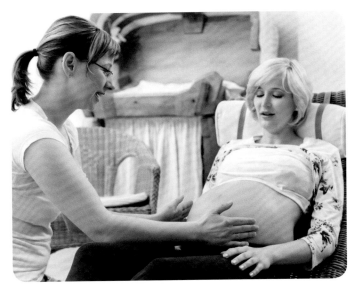

- Does the center screen patients and only allow low-risk births?
- Do they have backup arrangements with a hospital or physician in case of emergencies the facility cannot handle?
- How long do I stay after I give birth?
- If you or your baby require extra support, can the birthing center staff handle this or will you or your baby be transferred to another facility?
- Does my insurance cover the cost of this birthing center?

Birth Team

Remember, it is important that your relationship with your medical professional is built on trust and confidence. It is equally important that your medical professional convey warmth and a caring attitude toward you and the questions you ask. The more comfortable you are with your healthcare provider, the better and more enjoyable your birth experience will be.

Obstetrician

An obstetrician is a doctor trained to provide medical or surgical care in pregnancy, labor and birth. They are also trained to treat health problems and complications that can occur during pregnancy, birth and the postpartum period. The person you choose for your support and care should always take the time to listen to you, welcome your questions, and encourage you to have the safe and healthy pregnancy experience you desire.

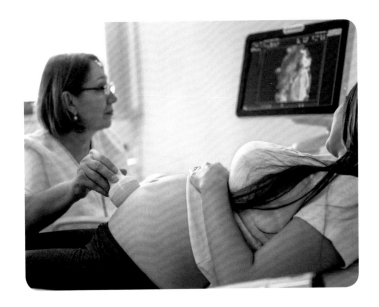

Family Medicine Doctor

Family doctors provide comprehensive healthcare for people of all ages, including pregnancy and birth. Most family care providers do not perform cesarean births. If you need a cesarean birth you would need to switch to an obstetrician's care.

Midwife

A midwife is a healthcare professional who provides compassionate, one-on-one attention and support during prenatal care, attends your labor, assists in the birth of your baby and provides postpartum care. Midwives become a collaborative partner with you, and understand that you are the central decision-maker in matters regarding your birth experience.

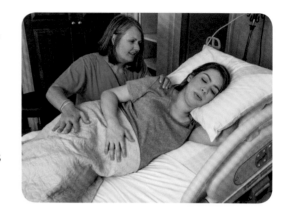

Some midwives are qualified healthcare providers who go through comprehensive training for certification. The practice and credentials related to midwifery differ throughout the United States.

There are different types of midwives:

Certified Nurse-Midwife (CNM)
An individual trained and licensed in both nursing and midwifery. Nurse-midwives possess at least a master's or doctoral degree from an accredited institution of higher education and are certified by the American College of Nurse Midwives.

Certified Professional Midwife (CPM)
An individual trained in midwifery who meets practice standards of the North American Registry of Midwives.

Direct-Entry Midwife (DEM)
An independent individual trained in midwifery through a variety of sources that can include: self-study, apprenticeship, a midwifery school or a college program.

Certified Midwife (CM)
An individual trained and certified in midwifery. Certified midwives possess at least a bachelor's degree from an accredited institution of higher education.

Lay Midwife
An individual who is not certified or licensed as a midwife but has been trained informally through self-study or apprenticeships.

Doula

A doula is a trained and experienced professional who provides continuous physical, emotional and informational support to you before, during and just after birth. A doula will typically meet you before your labor and stay with you throughout your labor and birth. A doula can help you with comfort measures and help you find the right solution for you. There are also doulas who provide emotional and practical support during the postpartum period.

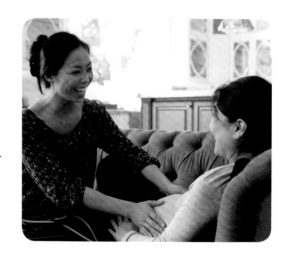

Studies have shown that when doulas attend birth, labors are shorter with fewer complications, babies are healthier and they breastfeed more easily. Evidence also shows that a postpartum doula can help with the transition that comes with a new baby. They can ease fears and help to promote balance for the entire family.

Labor Support Person

The support person you choose to have with you during your labor and birth can be invaluable so it makes sense to choose your support person carefully. For many people, this will be their partner or spouse. For others it might be a family member or friend. Whoever you pick should be aware that they are there to provide support and help, not just be a spectator or visit with other family members, while you are in labor.

10 things your support person can do to help you:

1 Emotional support
Keeping you informed on how you are progressing.

2 Reassurance
Telling you how they will support you and how much you mean to them.

3 Techniques taught in a class or online program
Willingness to breathe with you and help you stay relaxed between *contractions*.

4 Timing of contractions
Telling you how close together the contractions are and how long they may last.

5 Pressure points and massage
Guiding you with touch and massage to enable you to relax.

6 Understanding comfort measures
Positioning pillows all around you which will help with your ability to relax. Reminding you to change position frequently, moisten your lips and empty your bladder often.

7 Assessment of your relaxation needs
Suggesting new measures of relaxation or breathing techniques if you are having difficulty.

8 Crowd control
Making sure to know how many (and which) people you want in the room.

9 Updating family and friends
Providing information to your loved ones in the waiting room about your progress.

10 Support after the baby is born
Give you something to drink, get you a cool cloth for your face and celebrate you and your excellent work birthing.

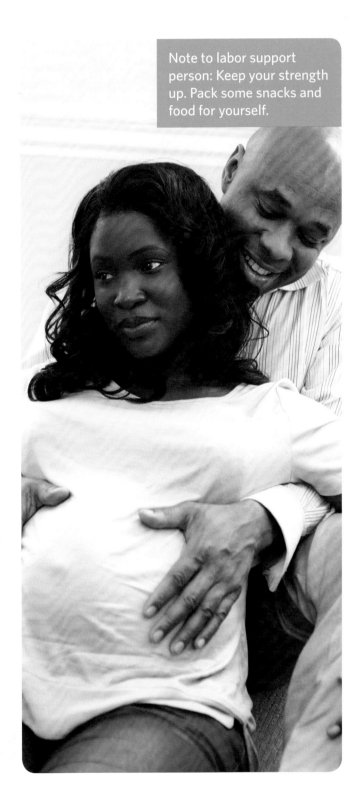

Note to labor support person: Keep your strength up. Pack some snacks and food for yourself.

Educators

Educational support from your childbirth educator or lactation consultant can relieve anxiety by helping you and your partner understand the process of labor and birth. It can also ensure the best possible start for you and your baby. Learning as much as you can about pregnancy and childbirth is a great way to get prepared for the big day.

With childbirth education you and your partner will learn:

- Pregnancy and labor are normal and healthy occurrences.
- To trust the process and not fight the contractions.
- Options available for managing labor and pain.
- To ask questions openly of the instructor and other class members.
- The importance of the partner in supporting the laboring person.

Birth Plan

You may have many questions and concerns as you get closer to your due date. Through childbirth education and your birth team, you will become more knowledgeable about the care options available to you. It is important to ask questions about what is happening during pregnancy and birth. When you ask questions and get the answers you need, you can make the best decisions for you and your baby.

The **"BRAIN"** acronym is a simple way to remember to ask about the benefits and risks of certain procedures, as well as to learn if you have other choices and time to think about your options. The acronym will also remind you to pay attention to your intuition, or "gut" feeling, about what is being suggested to you. You may find it helpful to use this guide when you meet your healthcare provider. In fact, you may find this a lifetime tool to help with decision-making.

Many decisions are made during labor and birth. Creating a birth plan ahead of time will help you think about what you hope will take place. You may want to write an outline of what you would like to happen. This can include decisions like which pain relief measures you would like, who you want in the room with you, and whether you want your partner to cut the *umbilical cord*. Add things that would enhance your experience and make you comfortable. A plan can help make your desires clear to everyone involved. Discuss your expectations with your birth team during your pregnancy in order to reduce surprises and disappointments later.

Informed Consent Questions for Labor and Birth		
	BENEFITS	• How will this help my labor? • How will this help my baby? • How will this help me?
• What is the procedure? • Why is it suggested? • What are my other options? • How could this affect my labor, my baby and me? • Do we have time to think it over? • What would happen if we do nothing? • Is this an emergency?	**R**ISKS	• How will this affect my labor? • How will this affect my baby? • How will this affect me?
	ALTERNATIVES	• What are my other options?
	INTUITION	• What does my gut say?
	NEED TIME	• I need time to think this decision through. • I need a private moment to talk with my family. • I would like to wait for now.

Communication

It is essential for you and your partner to open the lines of communication and share your feelings now, before your baby is born. There may be issues that both you and your support person are concerned about and many fears that you may be keeping from one another.

Your partner may have some of the following fears and concerns:

- Will labor be safe?
- Do I have what it takes to be a good parent?
- How can I be a good support person when I am afraid to see my partner in pain?
- How am I going to react when our baby is born? Will I pass out or be sick?
- Am I making enough money to support another family member?
- Will we have time together once our baby is born?

You may have some of the following fears and concerns:

- Will our baby be healthy?
- Am I going to be able to tolerate labor?
- I am afraid of needles and being in pain.
- Will I be a good parent?
- Will my partner still find me attractive after I give birth to our baby?
- Am I going to love this child at first sight?
- Will I work outside the home after the baby arrives?

These are all valid concerns and fears that you both may have and you might not talk about them. You may find comfort in discussing your worries and concerns openly. It will also allow you to speak more freely and openly with one another once your baby is born. Your baby will change your lives. Working on your communication skills now will help to keep the experience ahead of you a positive one and will continue to be important once your baby is born. You may find that working together to improve your communication skills better, brings you closer than ever before.

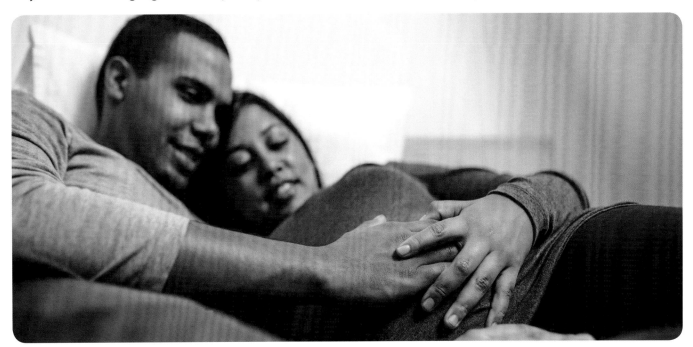

Selecting a Healthcare Provider for Your Baby

One thing you can think about before your admission to the hospital is who will take care of your baby after their birth. Start looking around as early in your pregnancy as possible. Your decision may largely depend on your insurance carrier. Talk to your friends. Ask who they use for their children and if they are happy with that healthcare provider. A lot of pediatricians and family care physicians will set appointments with you so that you can interview them. Consider choosing a healthcare provider for your newborn that is located close to you.

Questions to ask when interviewing a healthcare provider:

- What is their approach to health/wellness/sickness/preventive care?
- What is their perspective on breastfeeding, immunizations, or circumcision?
- What is the cost of a well-baby visit and is it covered by my insurance?
- Office hours – are there weekend and evening hours?
- Is there a sick room set up for children who are not feeling well?

Also investigate:

- Does the healthcare provider's personality match yours?
- Do they listen to you?
- How does the office run?
- How does the staff treat you?
- Is the office clean?

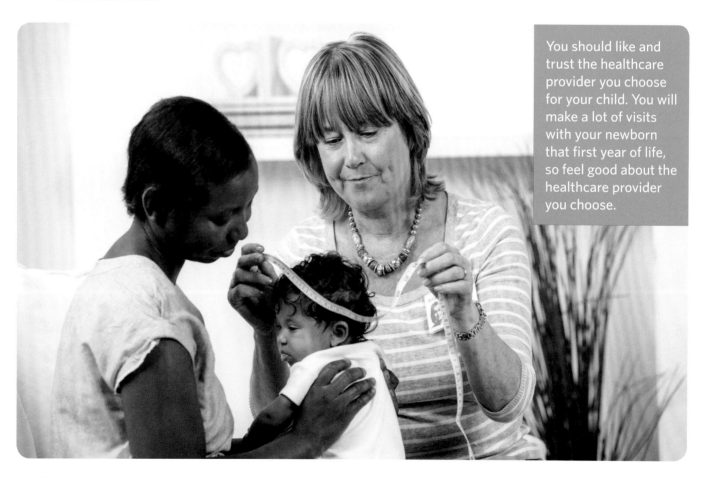

You should like and trust the healthcare provider you choose for your child. You will make a lot of visits with your newborn that first year of life, so feel good about the healthcare provider you choose.

Find supporting tools and videos in YoMingo.

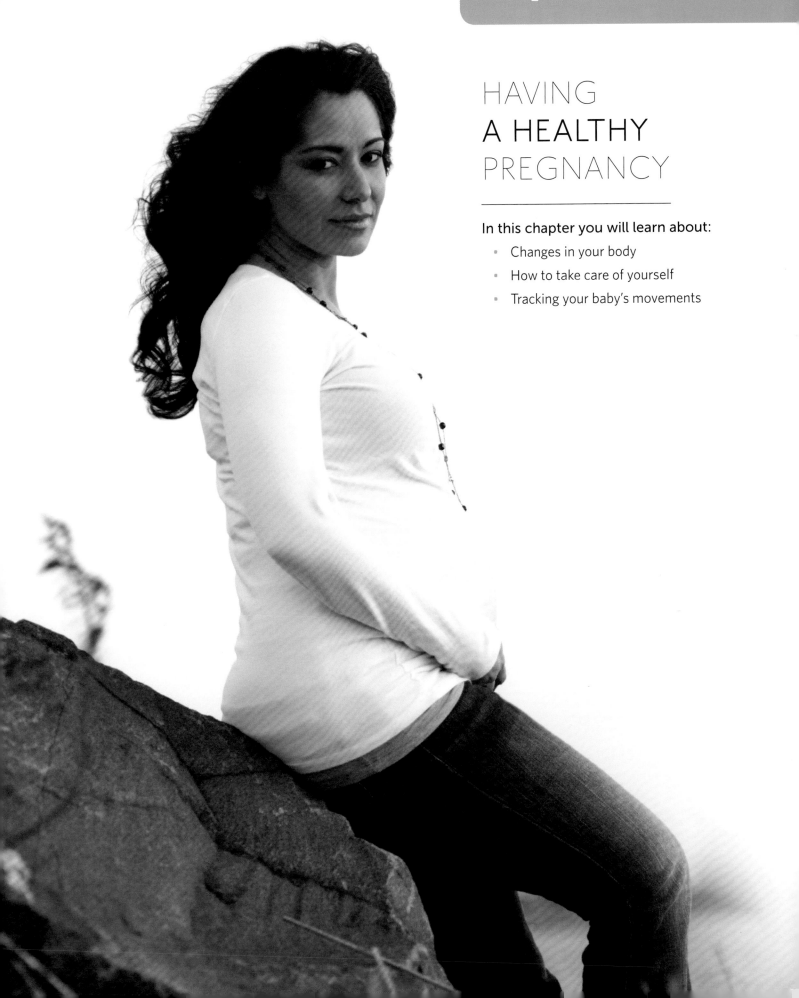

Chapter 2

HAVING A HEALTHY PREGNANCY

In this chapter you will learn about:

- Changes in your body
- How to take care of yourself
- Tracking your baby's movements

Activity and Health

Making healthy decisions during your pregnancy is essential not only for yourself but also for your growing baby. Keeping yourself fit and strong, making good choices in nutrition, and keeping your appointments with your healthcare provider are all necessary for a healthy pregnancy.

Physical Activity

Being active is beneficial both for you and for your baby's future health. Few people have activity restrictions during pregnancy but check with your healthcare provider before starting any exercise program.

Here are some benefits you may enjoy from staying active:

- Improved energy level.
- Improved endurance to better cope with labor and birth.
- Easier recovery after birth and return to pre-pregnancy fitness.
- Better cardiovascular health.
- Better circulation and less swelling.
- Improved muscle tone.
- Improved sleep.
- Better digestion with less constipation.
- Reduced backaches and muscle/joint soreness.
- Fewer emotional ups and downs.
- Reduced risk of gestational diabetes and preeclampsia.

Nutrition

During your second and third *trimesters* of pregnancy, you need a few extra calories a day to stay healthy and help your baby grow. One extra snack a day should fill the need. For example, have an apple with some peanut butter or a pear with a small piece of cheese as an afternoon snack.

Healthy eating plays an essential role in a healthy pregnancy. Try to eat foods from a variety of sources in order to get all the vitamins, minerals and nutrients you and your developing baby need. Eating well can help you feel better, give you more energy, and help you gain a healthy amount of weight. It will also contribute to your baby's growth and development. You should aim for 3 meals a day with healthy snacks in between.

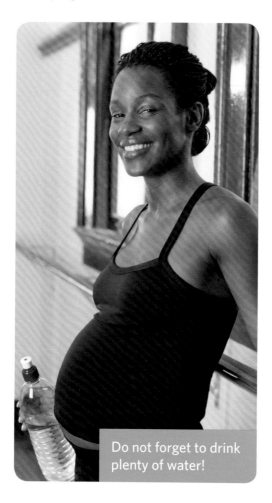

Do not forget to drink plenty of water!

Snacks to grab on the go!

- Pre-washed vegetables (carrots, cauliflower and broccoli)
- Small boxes of raisins
- Low-fat cottage cheese
- Low-fat yogurt
- Mixed vegetable juice or fruit juice
- Trail mix (raisins, dried fruit, nuts and seeds)
- Low-fat cheese

Extra calories for extra babies

Increase your daily intake:

For Twins:
- First Trimester — add 300 calories
- Second Trimester — add 680 calories
- Third Trimester — add 900 calories

For Triplets:
- First Trimester — add 450 calories
- Second Trimester — add 1,020 calories
- Third Trimester — add 1,350 calories

 Find supporting tools and videos in YoMingo.

Grains

Include grain products as part of your daily diet. Foods such as bread, rice and pasta are considered grains. Try to choose "whole grain" products that are lower in fat, sugar and salt.

Milk and Milk Alternatives

Drink skim, 1% or 2% milk every day and choose low-fat varieties of yogurt and cheese. Milk and milk alternatives are good for your growing baby because they will give you the high-quality protein, calcium and vitamin D you need but with less fat and calories. Drink fortified soy beverages if you do not drink cow's milk.

Meat and Meat Alternatives

Eating meat and meat alternatives each day will also help you and your baby stay healthy. Choose lean meats and meat alternatives such as dried peas, beans, tofu and lentils that are made with little or no added fat or salt. Fish is a healthy source of protein; try to eat it 2 to 3 times each week.

Fruits and Vegetables

Make half your plate fruits and vegetables. Eating colorful fruits and vegetables is important because they provide vitamins and minerals and most are low in calories. Vary your veggies. Try adding fresh, frozen or canned vegetables to salads, sides and main dishes. Choose a variety of colorful vegetables prepared in healthful ways: steamed, sautéed, roasted or raw.

Supplements

Take a prenatal vitamin every day that contains appropriate amounts of folic acid and iron. Folic acid is a B vitamin that protects your baby from birth defects of the spine and brain, also known as neural tube defects. When taking supplements, more is not better. You need just 0.4 to 0.8 mg of folic acid daily. You can get this amount from vitamins and fortified foods. Foods rich in folate are eggs, lentils, spinach, asparagus and oranges, as well as foods fortified with folic acid (such as white flour, bread or enriched pasta). A healthcare provider can help you find a prenatal vitamin that is right for you.

Raw Fish and Sushi	Raw fish and raw shellfish (sushi containing raw fish and oysters), smoked fish.
Undercooked Meat	Undercooked meat, poultry, hot dogs, deli meat.
Undercooked Eggs	Raw or lightly cooked eggs and foods containing them.
Alcohol	No amount of alcohol is safe during pregnancy.
Refrigerated Patés	Refrigerated patés and meat spreads.
Raw Sprouts	Raw sprouts (alfalfa sprouts).
Certain Types of Cooked Fish	Fish with high mercury content such as shark, tilefish, mackerel and swordfish.
Unpasteurized Products	Unpasteurized milk, milk products and juices (apple cider). Also, unpasteurized and pasteurized soft cheeses (feta, Brie, Camembert and blue-veined cheeses).

Emotional Health

Pregnancy is a time of enormous change. The hormonal changes within your body during pregnancy can trigger different emotions. Emotional changes such as joy and excitement, or even fear and panic, are all common during pregnancy. Emotional changes during and after pregnancy are easier to manage when you take care of yourself by doing the following:

- Get enough sleep and eat well-balanced meals.
- Exercise before and after the birth of your baby.
- Talk to friends and family for support.
- Discuss any symptoms or concerns with your healthcare provider.
- Attend support groups or new parent groups.

Oral Health

Maintain good oral health and continue to attend regular dental checkups during pregnancy. Remember to tell your dentist that you are pregnant. Brush your teeth twice daily for 2 minutes and do not forget to floss.

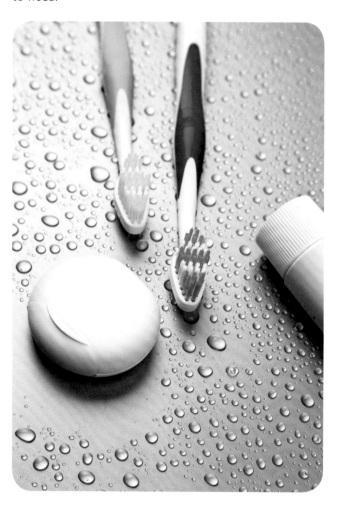

Smoking

Smoking should be avoided during pregnancy. Even secondhand smoke contains the same 4,000 chemicals a smoker would inhale. More than 40 of those chemicals are known to cause cancer.

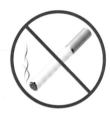

Smoking and secondhand smoke can have the following negative effects:

- Decreased oxygen to your baby.
- Increased risk of miscarriage.
- Complications during birth.
- Increased incidences of chest and ear infections, as well as asthma, in babies.
- Low birth weight.
- Higher risk of Sudden Infant Death Syndrome (SIDS).

Alcohol

There is no amount of alcohol that is safe during pregnancy. As soon as you know you are pregnant, avoid all alcoholic drinks such as beer, wine, champagne, liquors, cocktails and coolers. Drinking alcohol during pregnancy puts your baby at many risks including brain damage and birth defects, also known as Fetal Alcohol Syndrome (FAS).

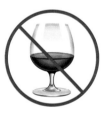

Discomforts of Pregnancy

There are many changes and discomforts that occur throughout your pregnancy. Although every person's pregnancy is different, there are some similarities in the aches and pains that you may encounter. Many of these physical and emotional changes are due to *hormones*.

This illustration shows the physical changes that will occur in your body during pregnancy.

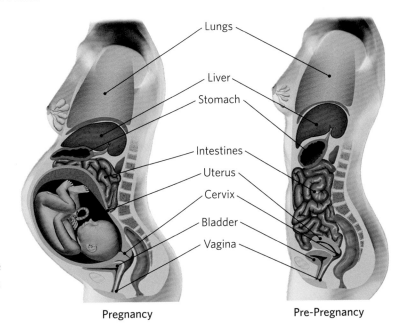

Lungs
Liver
Stomach
Intestines
Uterus
Cervix
Bladder
Vagina

Pregnancy   Pre-Pregnancy

Nausea and Vomiting

It is very common for you to have nausea and vomiting during pregnancy. This is also called "morning sickness" but it can happen at any time of the day. Nausea and vomiting are thought to be due to the hormones of pregnancy. It usually ends by 16 weeks, but some people continue to have it throughout their pregnancy.

Things that may help with nausea and vomiting:

- Eat small, frequent meals.
- Drink small amounts of liquids frequently during the day but not with meals.
- Eat crackers or dry toast.
- Get out of bed slowly.
- Do not lie down right after eating.
- Try to stay hydrated.

Shortness of Breath

As your baby grows, they put pressure on your internal organs and *diaphragm*. Your lungs do not have as much room to expand as they did before pregnancy. You will breathe easier once your baby descends into the *pelvis*.

If shortness of breath is a problem for you:

- Avoid sleeping flat on your back. Lying on your side at night is usually more comfortable.
- Use pillows all around you — between your legs and behind your back.
- Prop yourself up at night instead of lying flat.
- Sleep in a recliner with pillows surrounding you.
- Slow down when climbing stairs.

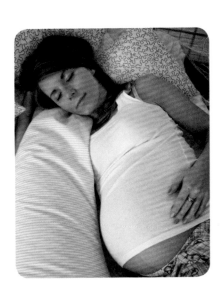

Swelling

You may experience swelling of the feet and legs toward the end of your pregnancy. With the added weight of pregnancy, your circulation is slower at returning fluid to the heart, especially from way down at your feet. If you have excessive swelling of your legs, notify your healthcare provider. Also notify them if you have swelling in your hands and face, as this may signal something more serious, such as high blood pressure.

Try the following to relieve swelling:

- Elevate your legs whenever possible.
- Place pillows between your legs when lying down.
- Try not to cross your legs when sitting.
- Lie on your side when sleeping or resting.
- Drink plenty of water.
- Have some daily physical activity, such as swimming and walking.

> Excessive swelling could be a sign of preeclampsia of pregnancy. It is a condition related to pregnancy and the postpartum period. Preeclampsia needs medical attention.

Preeclampsia

Preeclampsia is a disorder that occurs only during pregnancy, typically after 20 weeks. It can also appear up to 6 weeks postpartum. This condition can affect both you and your baby. Proper prenatal care is essential to diagnose and manage preeclampsia. At least 5 to 8 percent of all pregnant people have this condition.

Signs and symptoms:

- High blood pressure.
- Protein in your urine.
- Swelling.
- Headache not relieved by acetaminophen.
- Nausea or vomiting.
- Pain in your stomach area and/or shoulder pain.
- Lower back pain.
- Sudden weight gain.
- Changes in your vision.
- Hyperreflexia – your reflexes are strong and overreactive.
- Shortness of breath, anxiety.

Please know that it is possible to have preeclampsia and not have any symptoms. That is why it is so important not to miss any prenatal and postpartum appointments.

Find supporting tools and videos in YoMingo.

Nasal Congestion

Nasal congestion is a very common problem. Your nose may feel stuffy and you may experience nosebleeds during pregnancy. Your blood volume increases during pregnancy which affects the membranes inside your nose and causes them to swell. Sometimes they may even feel very dry and raw, which causes the bleeding.

Some tips to reduce nasal congestion:

- Try saline nose drops or sprays.
- Use a cool mist humidifier in your home.
- Avoid medicated nose drops or sprays.

Heartburn

Your stomach is also affected by your growing baby — it does not have the capacity to hold as much food as it did before you were pregnant. Acid from your stomach rises up into the esophagus and causes a burning sensation. You may be uncomfortable when trying to rest or sleep due to this acid reflux in the chest or even a dry cough.

The following suggestions may help with your discomfort:

- Eat small, frequent meals during the day.
- Avoid eating near bedtime.
- Drink fluids between meals instead of during meals.
- Wear loose clothing.
- Stay upright after eating.
- Avoid spicy and fatty foods.
- Avoid coffee, carbonated drinks and chocolate.
- Eat slowly and chew your food well.
- Use pillows to prop yourself up at night if acid reflux is a problem.

Backache

Probably one of the most common problems in pregnancy, and the one that frequently worsens as pregnancy progresses, is backache. Your pregnancy affects your posture and how you walk, especially at the end of the day when you are tired. The "pregnancy waddle" is caused by compensating for the extra weight you are carrying out front by arching and curving your back inward.

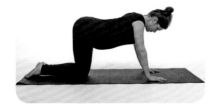

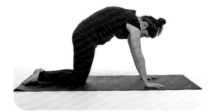

Helpful suggestions for back discomfort:

- Remind yourself to walk with your back straight and avoid the "waddle."
- Take breaks throughout the day and rest your back.
- Wear low, rubber-soled shoes.
- Place a small pillow or rolled towel in the lower part of your back when sitting down or driving your car.
- Exercise to strengthen your back and abdominal muscles.
- Avoid lifting anything heavy. Never bend at the waist to lift — always bend at the knees, keeping your back straight.
- When getting out of bed in the morning, roll onto your side first and push yourself up to a sitting position. Never sit straight up from lying on your back.

A simple back exercise, as shown, is very helpful in relieving back discomfort.

Sciatica

Some women will experience this discomfort off and on during pregnancy. It causes tingling, numbness and/or pain affecting the buttocks, hips and thighs — usually on just one side. The enlarging *uterus* and growing baby put pressure on these nerves. Sometimes a simple change in position of the baby may help to alleviate the discomforts of sciatica. If you are troubled by these symptoms, talk to your healthcare provider.

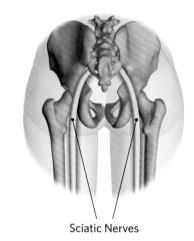

Sciatic Nerves

> The sciatic nerves branch from the lower back down the buttocks and legs to the feet. While sciatica may be bothersome and uncomfortable, please know this usually goes away after pregnancy.

Round Ligament Pain

The round ligaments attach each side of the uterus to the groin region. As the uterus grows, these fibrous ligaments stretch like a rubber band. Any sudden movement or position change can cause them to spasm or stretch, which can cause pain. Sometimes this discomfort, known as *round ligament pain*, can be very severe. You may be out for a walk and suddenly feel a sharp pain on one or both sides of your abdomen or groin. The pain can be constant or intermittent and sharp or aching. Resting and applying a heating pad on low setting may be helpful. A maternity belt can help support your uterus and lessen stress on these ligaments.

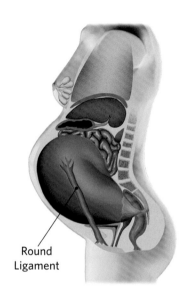

Round Ligament

> **Important:** If you have abdominal pain and it continues or becomes more intense, call your healthcare provider or go to the hospital immediately.

Loose and Aching Joints

You may feel as if your joints are loose, they pop or just feel achy. Cartilage is found between the joints. Hormones released toward the end of your pregnancy soften the cartilage joining the pubic bone in front of the pelvis. It allows the pelvis to expand 1 to 1 1/2 centimeters, enlarging the bony opening for the baby to pass through. This is not the only place that cartilage is found. It is up your back, between your spine, in your ankles and your toes. Some people even have a sense of achiness throughout their bodies.

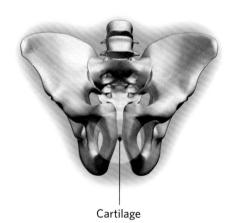

Cartilage

Hemorrhoids and Constipation

Hemorrhoids are common during pregnancy. They are enlarged veins at the opening of the rectum, which can become swollen, painful and itchy. It's possible they may bleed. Hemorrhoids can be internal as well as external.

If hemorrhoids and constipation are a problem for you, try these tips to provide relief:

- Eat a high-fiber diet (fruit, whole-grain cereal and raw vegetables).
- Drink plenty of water throughout the day.
- Incorporate a light exercise activity to your day, such as walking.
- Warm tub baths may be soothing.
- Do not give yourself an *enema* or take over-the-counter laxatives or suppositories.
- Ice packs and witch hazel pads may be applied directly to hemorrhoids.
- Report continued bleeding to your healthcare provider.

Frequent Urination

What may be a problem in the beginning of your pregnancy comes back full force in the last trimester. As the uterus grows it places a lot of pressure on the bladder — even more so when the baby descends into the pelvis. Every time you cough, sneeze or laugh too hard, you may pass a small amount of urine. It may help to do *Kegel exercises*.

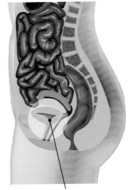 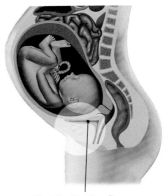

Bladder Before Pregnancy   Bladder During Pregnancy

Kegel exercises

Kegel exercises help you learn how to contract and relax the pelvic floor muscles. They are very beneficial exercises and easy to do. The Kegel can also help control urine leakage by strengthening some of the muscles that resist urine flow.

If you do not know how to relax these muscles, it may be more difficult for you to push effectively during birth. The exercise involves contracting the muscles around the *vagina* (as though stopping the flow of urine midstream) by squeezing the muscles tightly for a few seconds and then relaxing them. Squeeze and relax 10 times, at least 5 times daily. You can also do this exercise by slowly tightening the muscles from bottom to top as if going up an elevator — first floor through the fifth floor. Then slowly allow the muscles to relax by coming down the elevator. Learn about the different levels of tension and relaxation. An awareness of this exercise will help you to be more effective when pushing during the second stage of labor. This exercise is also beneficial postpartum to regain the loss of muscle tone around the vagina and urethra.

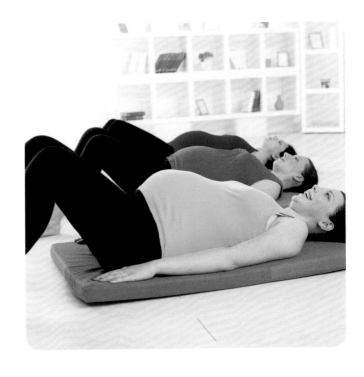

Breast Changes

During pregnancy you may notice your breasts getting larger and sometimes feeling tender. The nipple and the area around the nipple, known as the *areola*, enlarge and become darker in color. As they prepare for milk production, you may notice that the blood vessels of the breasts can be seen at the skin surface. Your breast may tingle with temperature change or touch. Sometimes *colostrum* will leak from your breasts during pregnancy. Do not be concerned if your breasts do not leak. It does not mean that you will be unable to produce milk. Some people have breasts that leak and some do not.

Guidelines for breast care:

- Wear a bra that provides firm support.
- Buy a bra that fits without pressing, binding or rubbing. You may need to buy a larger bra around the third or fourth month of pregnancy.
- You may be more comfortable wearing a bra at night if your breasts are large.
- Clean colostrum from your breasts using only warm water.
- If colostrum leakage is a problem, wear an absorbent breast pad in your bra and replace it when wet to avoid irritation or infection.

Skin Changes

You may notice that you have a dark line running up and down your abdomen. This is called *linea nigra* and is due to hormone changes that affect the skin's pigmentation. Some women will notice darkness around their nose or face. This is known as *chloasma*. Both of these will fade postpartum as the hormone levels get back to normal. Although these changes may be worrisome to you, they are not harmful and will not cause permanent scarring or damage to your skin. *Stretch marks* can be found not only on the abdomen but also on the breasts, thighs, buttocks and upper arms.

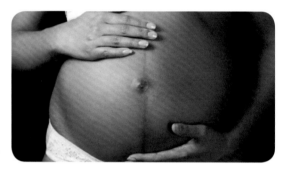

Linea Nigra

Fatigue and Insomnia

Fatigue and *insomnia* are common in the last trimester and may be frustrating to you. Rest as much as you can. LISTEN TO YOUR BODY. When it tells you that you are tired — REST. Anxiety can also play a role in insomnia.

Here are some things that may help with insomnia:

- Take a warm shower before bedtime — this may help to relax you.
- Read a good book before bed.
- Leave the bedroom where you are having difficulty sleeping. Sometimes a change of rooms will help.
- Make yourself as comfortable as possible with pillows.
- Avoid caffeinated beverages.
- Try using relaxation techniques.
- Avoid exercise immediately before bedtime.
- Do not take any over-the-counter medications without talking to your healthcare provider first! Whatever you take goes to the baby as well.

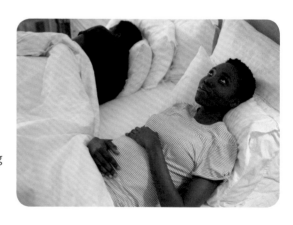

Leg Cramps

If you experience a leg cramp, try to straighten your leg and point your toes toward your head. You should feel immediate relief. This works better than rubbing your leg. You may need to stand on the affected leg to adequately stretch the muscle that is cramping. Proceed with caution, however, as sometimes you may lose the ability to stand on the leg that is cramping. Practice stretching exercises 2 to 3 times each day, especially before bedtime. This will help prevent leg cramps.

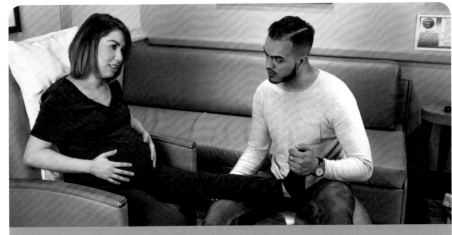

Your partner can help relieve a leg cramp by straightening your leg and pushing your toes toward your head.

Tracking Your Baby's Movement ↺

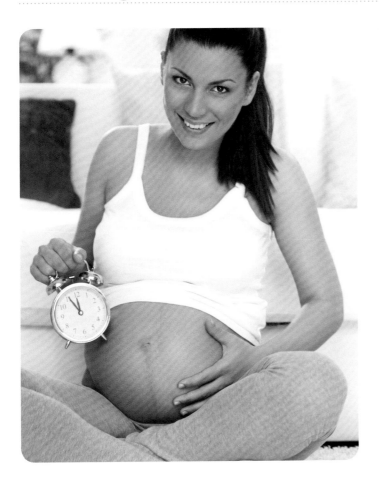

Your healthcare provider may have you monitor your baby's movements like this:

- Choose a time of day when your baby tends to be active.

- Make sure that you have eaten a snack and have had a cold drink of water recently.

- Sit quietly or lie on your side and try not to be distracted.

- Time how long it takes to feel 10 distinct movements, kicks, punches, swooshes and body movements.

- According to ACOG (American Congress of Obstetricians and Gynecologists), generally 10 movements in 2 hours is considered reassuring. If you feel fewer than 10, you should contact your healthcare provider. Remember, your baby's activity level will vary throughout the day, but you should feel your baby's movements throughout the day, every day.

↺ Find supporting tools and videos in YoMingo.

Warning Signs Which Need Immediate Attention:

Preterm Labor (3 or more weeks before your due date)

- Contractions – more than 4 occurring in an hour.
- Menstrual-like cramps – may come and go or be constant.
- Abdominal cramps – may occur with or without diarrhea.
- Low backache – comes and goes or is constant.
- Pelvic pressure – feels like the baby is pushing down.
- Change in vaginal discharge – a sudden increase in the amount or it may become more mucus-like, watery or slightly blood-tinged.
- Water breaks before 37 weeks.
  - Note how much fluid – small leak or big gush?
  - What color is the fluid?
  - If you are not sure if it is your water that has broken or if you passed urine, call your healthcare provider and get it checked right away.

Vaginal Bleeding (bright red vaginal bleeding is not normal) Note the following:

- Amount of bleeding.
- Presence of clots.

Abdominal Pain

- Seek immediate medical attention.

Decreased Fetal Movement

- Absence of movement or significant lessening of movement may be of concern; notify your healthcare provider immediately.
- See "Tracking Your Baby's Movement" on previous page.

Fever

- Notify your healthcare provider if you have a fever (temperature more than 100.4°F).

Headache

- Unusually severe and unrelieved with acetaminophen.
- Seeing spots or flashing lights.
- Other neurological symptoms – numbness, loss of vision, weakness, loss of balance, or speech difficulty.

Urinary Discomfort

- Frequent with small amounts.
- Painful urination.
- Blood-tinged urine.
- Pus in urine.

> If you experience any of the warning signs listed here or have other symptoms that you feel are not normal, get medical attention immediately.

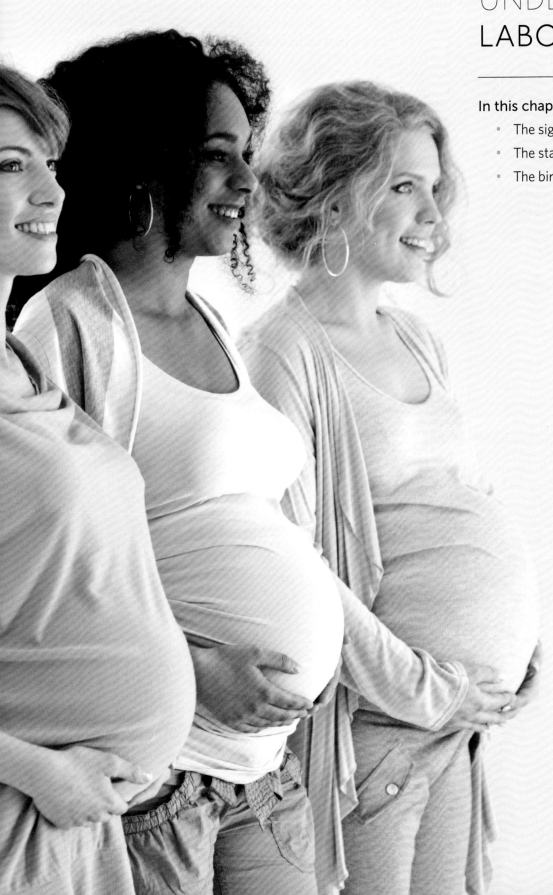

Chapter 3

UNDERSTANDING LABOR AND BIRTH

In this chapter you will learn about:

- The signs of labor
- The stages of labor
- The birth of your baby

Labor Terms

Uterine muscle cells work like other muscle cells in your body to tighten or contract the muscle. During labor, uterine muscles start contracting at the top of the uterus, known as the *fundus*. This causes tightening and pressure, which moves from the top of the uterus to the bottom in a wave-like fashion. These contractions force your baby to move downward through your pelvis and out of the cervical opening into the vagina, or birth canal. Your body will manage your labor through a well-coordinated process. Your contractions will repeat in shorter intervals and increase in intensity until your baby is born.

The start of labor occurs when the contractions create changes to the *cervix*. It is possible for you to have many episodes of contractions prior to the onset of labor. The average time of labor is about 12 to 18 hours for the first baby, but everyone's experience is different. Your labor could be as short as 4 hours or as long as 24 hours or more. Remember, it is important to manage your expectations.

Bag of Waters or Amniotic Sac

You never know where you are going to be or when your labor will begin. It may start with contractions or with your water breaking. The medical term for your water breaking is "ruptured membranes." This is when the sac that contains the *amniotic fluid* around your baby leaks or breaks open completely. If you think your water has broken, your healthcare provider may want to know the time your water broke, what color it is, the odor and the amount.

The sac of amniotic fluid serves these purposes:

- Acts as a cushion for the baby.
- Keeps the environment and temperature stable for the growing baby.
- Keeps bacteria from entering where the baby is growing and developing.

Mucous Plug

You may remember the hormonal changes that made you moody or teary at the beginning of your pregnancy. One of the benefits of those early hormone surges was the development of what is known as the *mucous plug*. As the cervix softens, the plug may be dislodged. It is a very thick, stringy piece of mucus that may not always be noticed. Once the mucous plug is expelled, it could be moments or days until labor begins. It could, however, be one of the signs of pre-labor. The plug blocks the long cervix and helps to prevent bacteria from getting into the uterus. The cervix has a rich blood supply, so as the mucus passes through the cervix it may become blood-tinged. This is called *bloody show*.

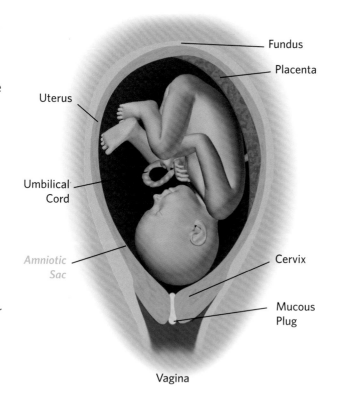

Placenta

The *placenta* is a remarkable organ that is only present during pregnancy. Not only does it produce hormones to support your pregnancy, but it also provides the oxygen and nutrients that your growing baby needs and removes the waste products from your baby's blood. The placenta develops on the wall of the uterus and the umbilical cord extends from it, connecting you to your baby. Once your baby has been born, the placenta's purpose is completed and it will be expelled. Depending on your health during pregnancy, your placenta may be sent to a pathology lab for further inspection, or it may simply be discarded.

Labor Hormones

No one really knows or understands why, when or how labor begins. What healthcare providers do know is that there are chemicals produced by the body known as *prostaglandins*, which cause softening and thinning of the cervix toward the end of the third trimester. When your body is ready to give birth to your baby, large quantities of prostaglandins are released. An increase in the sensitivity of *oxytocin* receptors in the uterus stimulates contractions once labor has begun.

Braxton Hicks Contractions

Throughout most of your pregnancy, the uterine muscles commonly contract from time to time. These contractions are often painless, irregular in frequency and mild in intensity. Many people describe them as a "balling up" sensation.

These contractions are the way your uterine muscles stay in shape and practice for the upcoming labor. Sometimes it is difficult to tell the difference between labor and *Braxton Hicks contractions*.

Lightening

Earlier in your pregnancy, your fundus (top of the uterus) was positioned high in your abdomen, just underneath your breasts. As your baby's birth nears, the fundus will drop 2 to 3 inches away from your ribs. This process is called *lightening*. It can occur weeks before the onset of labor or anytime right up to when labor begins. Many people describe it as increased pressure in the pelvic area. This pressure results from the baby's head settling into the bony pelvis. It is now easier for you to breathe, but you may feel more pressure on your bladder, and you may be making more trips to the bathroom.

Effacement

After prostaglandins soften your cervix, they further prepare your body for birth by the *effacement*, or thinning out, of your cervix. The cervix is normally 1 $\frac{1}{2}$ to 2 inches long but will become paper-thin as it expands and pulls over your baby's head.

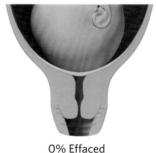 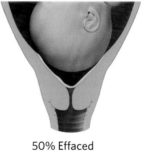 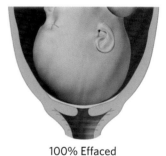

| 0% Effaced | 50% Effaced | 100% Effaced |

Dilation

Dilation is when the cervix opens gradually to allow your baby to pass through into the birth canal. Dilation is measured in centimeters, from 0 to 10. Both effacement and dilation are estimated during a vaginal exam and are subjective measurements.

One way to help you visualize these changes is for you to think about a long neck bottle. If you hold it upside down, you can think of it as your cervix. It has a very long, thick neck. Compare this image to a wide mouth jar held upside down. The neck of the jar is thinned out and its opening measures about 10 centimeters. This is a strange analogy but a great way for you to visualize exactly how the process of labor changes the cervix.

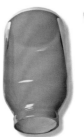 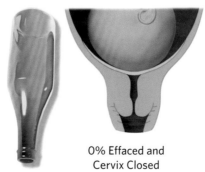 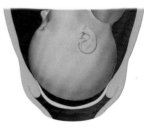

0% Effaced and Cervix Closed

100% Effaced and Cervix Completely Dilated (10 cm)

Dilation Chart

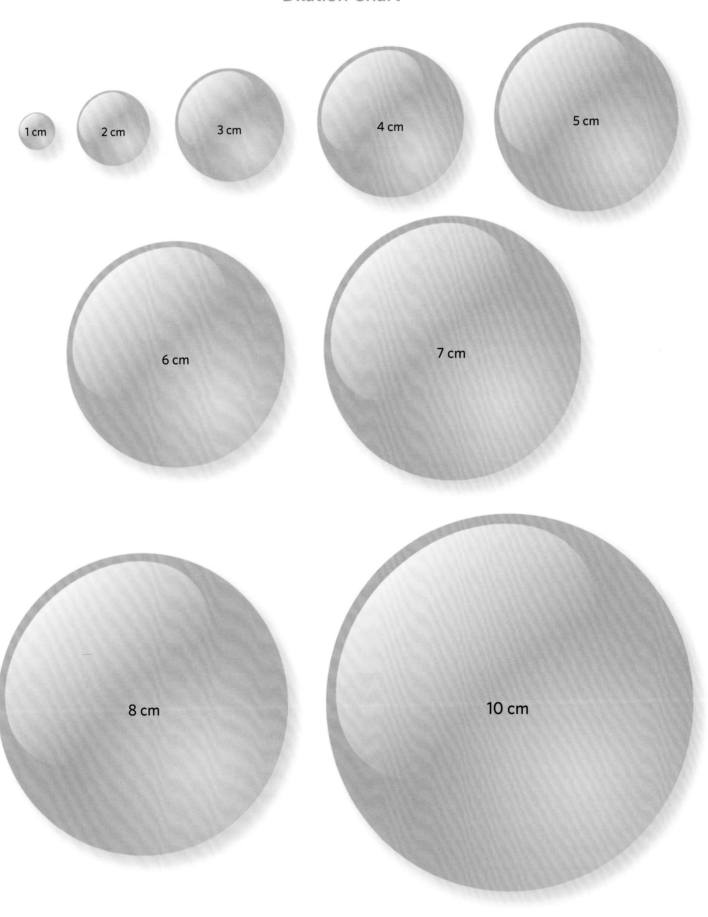

1 cm

2 cm

3 cm

4 cm

5 cm

6 cm

7 cm

8 cm

10 cm

Station

The relationship of the top of the baby's head or presenting part to the spines of your pelvic bones is known as *station*. During a vaginal exam your healthcare provider can feel 2 bony prominences through your vaginal wall. These are known as the ischial spines. If the baby's head is above the ischial spines, the station is a negative number (–). Below the spines it is a positive number (+) as shown in the diagram. For example, +2 station means the head is 2 centimeters below the spines.

> When the fetal head is at the level of the bony spine landmark, it is called 0 (zero) station.

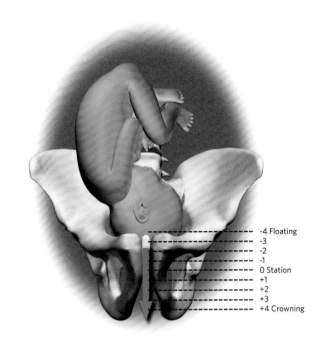

-4 Floating
-3
-2
-1
0 Station
+1
+2
+3
+4 Crowning

Common Questions About Labor

Am I Really in Labor?

This may be one of your biggest concerns while you are pregnant. As you get closer to your due date, it is important for you to understand the difference between labor contractions and practice labor contractions.

Labor contractions

- Contractions occur at regular intervals.
- Intensity of contractions increases.
- Intervals between contractions shorten.
- Discomfort in back and/or lower abdomen.
- Discomfort does not stop with walking.
- Cervix dilates.

Braxton Hicks contractions

- Contractions occur at irregular intervals.
- Intensity relatively unchanged.
- Intervals between contractions do not get shorter.
- Discomfort primarily in lower abdomen.
- Discomfort frequently relieved with walking.
- Cervix does not dilate.

How Do I Time Contractions?

To time contractions, 2 specific characteristics of the contraction are recorded — frequency and duration.

Frequency: Time from the start of 1 contraction to the start of the following contraction.

Duration: Time from the start of 1 contraction to the end of that same contraction.

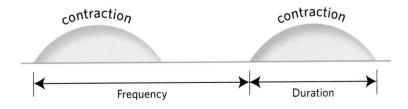

contraction   contraction

Frequency   Duration

 Find supporting tools and videos in YoMingo.

When Should I Go to the Hospital?

Ask your healthcare provider this question, because the answer may vary depending on your personal circumstances. The most important thing is to listen to your instincts and go when you feel you need to go.

Remember, there are no two labors exactly alike, so your healthcare provider might instruct you differently from other expecting parents. Each pregnancy may have unique issues. LISTEN TO YOUR BODY.

Go to the hospital when:

- Your water breaks with a gush or continues to leak.
- Your contractions are consistent and 5 minutes apart for at least an hour. This number may change if you are further than 30 minutes away from your hospital.
- Your healthcare provider recommends you go.
- Or you feel you need to go.

Contractions – Report the following information about your contractions. Are they:

- Growing more intense?
- Following a regular pattern?
- Lasting longer?
- Becoming closer together?

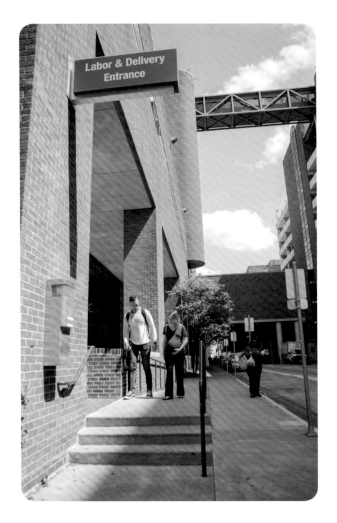

What Factors Affect My Labor?

There are many factors that will determine how long your labor will last or how long it takes to go from one stage to the next.

The blending of the following factors can affect your progress in labor:

- Position of your baby's head.
- Size of your baby.
- *Presentation* of your baby. Cephalic or vertex (head first), *breech* (feet or buttocks first) or *transverse lie* (arm or chest first).
- Size and shape of your pelvis.
- Your physical and emotional state.
- The effectiveness of the contractions in dilating the cervix.
- Your labor partner and the support they provide.
- Medications or *anesthesia* administered.

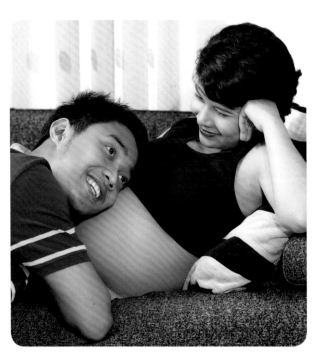

Pre-Labor

Pre-labor are the changes that occur during the days before you give birth. You may experience the nesting instinct and feel like you have more energy. Remember that this is also a time to rest and save your energy for birth. Pre-labor is your body's way of preparing for the event of labor.

Emotions and reactions

- Combination of excitement and anxiety.
- Burst of energy or the nesting instinct.
- You want to make contact with friends and family.

Physical changes

- More episodes of Braxton Hicks contractions.
- Increased vaginal discharge.
- Possible loss of mucous plug.
- Increased pressure on pelvic floor.
- Some nausea and diarrhea.
- Premenstrual symptoms.

Comfort measures

- Continue with normal daily activities.
- Focus on taking more naps — REST!
- Practice relaxation and breathing techniques with your support person.
- Practice working together as a team with your support person.
- Finish last-minute details and make necessary arrangements.
- Have your hospital bag packed and ready to go.

Role of support person

- Help with last-minute arrangements.
- Make sure you both get the proper rest needed.
- Share your feelings, fears and concerns with your labor partner. If you talk about your fears, they may not be so scary.

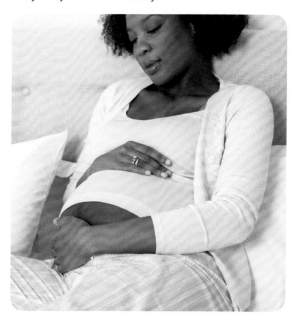

Stages of Labor

The labor process is unique for every family. The information about the duration and frequency of contractions in each stage of labor is an average. It is more important that you listen to and trust your own body about how your labor is progressing. There are 3 stages of labor. During each stage, many changes are occurring within your body.

First Stage of Labor

Within the first stage of labor there are 3 phases:

- Early labor
- Active labor
- Transition

The first stage occurs from the time labor begins until the cervix is completely dilated.

Second Stage of Labor

The second stage of labor is from complete cervical dilation until the birth of your baby.

Third Stage of Labor

The third stage of labor is from the birth of your baby until the placenta detaches from the uterine wall and is expelled through the vagina.

Find supporting tools and videos in YoMingo.

First Stage of Labor

The first stage begins with the onset of labor and ends when the cervix is completely dilated (10 centimeters). The average duration for this stage for people having their first child (*primipara*) is 6 to 12 hours, but it can last as long as 20 hours. For people having their second or third baby (*multipara*), this stage may be shorter. The first stage of labor is usually the longest because there are many phases within this stage. There are 3 phases within the first stage of labor: The early or latent labor, active labor and transition.

Early Labor

Emotions and reactions

- Excitement; eagerness to begin; anticipation of labor experience.
- Thoughts of fear and anxiety: There is no turning back! This is it. Do I remember everything that I learned in class?
- Talkative; very social; want conversation and interaction with partner.
- Fully aware of surroundings; interested in what is going on; eager to report symptoms.

Physical changes

- Contractions are typically mild and somewhat irregular, but progressively stronger and closer together.
- Contractions may start out every 15 to 20 minutes apart and eventually become 5 minutes apart, lasting from 40 to 60 seconds as you reach the end of early labor.
- Contractions may be experienced as an aching or low backache, menstrual-type cramps, pressure or tightening in the pubic area.
- The amniotic sac may rupture; also a pink mucous vaginal discharge could be evident, commonly known as "show."

Comfort measures

- It is important to balance rest and light activity at this stage.
- Light activity, such as walking, can be helpful.
- Eat and drink fluids as desired.
- Use slow, relaxed breathing as long as you find it works for you.
- Begin comfort measures as your contractions become stronger.

Role of support person

- It is important to give words of encouragement during labor. Help balance light activity and rest.
- Time the contractions and write them down to report to the healthcare provider.
- Provide diversions such as music, playing cards or watching a good movie.
- Be aware of how they are reacting to their contractions; check for relaxation and breathing.
- Listen actively; offer praise.
- Contact your healthcare provider and your birthing facility.
- Check the weather and have the car ready or a ride available.

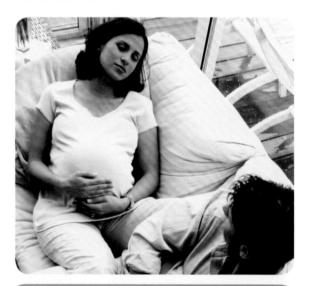

Early labor in a snapshot:
- Cervix dilates from closed to 6 centimeters.
- Contractions are from 5 to 15 minutes apart.
- Contractions last from 40 to 60 seconds.
- Phase can last from 6 to 8 hours on average.

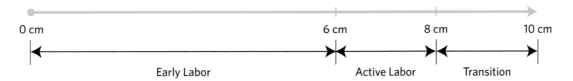

0 cm   6 cm   8 cm   10 cm

Early Labor   Active Labor   Transition

Early Labor

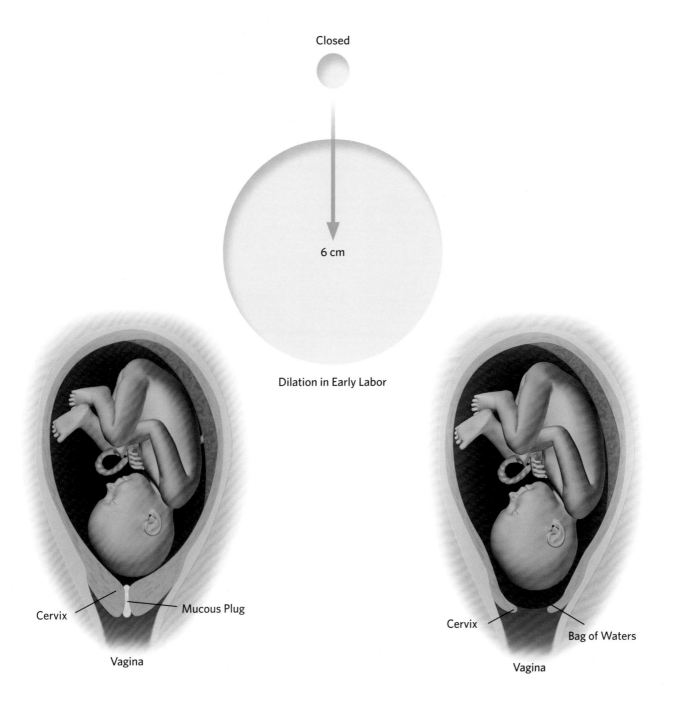

Closed

6 cm

Dilation in Early Labor

Cervix   Mucous Plug

Vagina

Cervix

Bag of Waters

Vagina

Emotions and reactions

- No longer social; very much involved in the work of labor.
- More serious and less talkative; concentrate and focus on relaxation techniques that work.
- Selectively attentive.
- May have a hard time understanding conversation during contractions.
- Desires and needs companionship from support person.

Physical changes

- Contractions become progressively stronger and closer together — 2 to 4 minutes apart and lasting 45 to 60 seconds in duration.
- Longer peaks in contractions and increasingly uncomfortable.
- Pressure or tightening in pubic area.
- May experience dry mouth and perspiration.
- May become more focused; find it hard to rest and relax.
- May experience nausea and vomiting.
- May appear pale or flushed.

Comfort measures

- Do not fight the contractions; allow them to do their job.
- Continue with breathing and relaxation techniques that work for you.
- Add abdominal massage with breathing techniques.
- Concentrate on a focal point during contractions. This will help distract from the discomfort of labor.
- A shower or bath can be very comforting.
- Changing positions regularly will help the baby to move through your pelvis. Try to stay out of bed unless you need to rest or for an exam by your nurse or healthcare provider.

Role of support person

- Give all of your attention. Breathe together.
- Offer verbal support and encouragement.
- Offer a cool, damp washcloth.
- Encourage hourly trips to the bathroom to keep bladder empty.
- Keep their lips moist with petroleum-free balm.
- Offer ice chips and light snacks.
- Surround them with pillows to keep them comfortable and relaxed.
- Apply pressure to their lower back, if needed.
- Use touch, massage and relaxation techniques.
- Encourage frequent position changes.

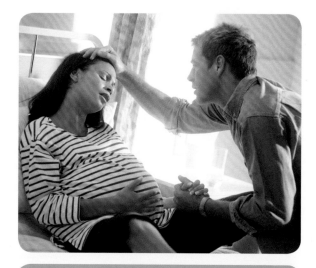

Active labor in a snapshot:

- Cervix dilates from 6 to 8 centimeters.
- Contractions range from 2 to 4 minutes apart.
- Contractions last from 45 to 60 seconds.
- Phase can last from 4 to 6 hours on average.

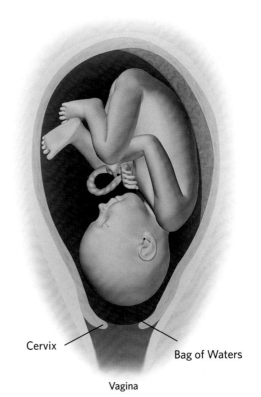

Cervix — Bag of Waters

Vagina

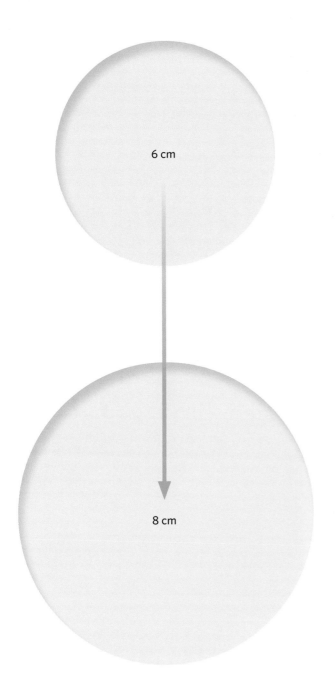

6 cm

8 cm

Dilation in Active Labor

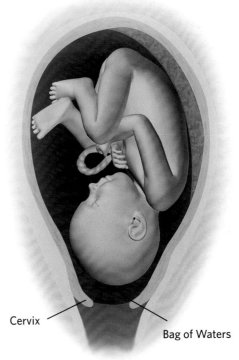

Cervix — Bag of Waters

Vagina

Transition

Emotions and reactions

- Rely on partner for support.
- May express intense emotions.
- May feel out of control and cry.
- May need labor partner for help with breathing routine.
- May fall asleep between contractions.
- May be less aware of surroundings.
- Focus is very inward.

Physical changes

- Long and strong contractions that peak very quickly or double peak and are intense.
- Contractions every 1 ½ to 2 minutes, lasting 60 to 90 seconds.
- May experience rectal pressure or urge to *bear down*.
- Increased bloody show.
- Severe low backache.
- Nausea, vomiting, hiccuping, belching, and passing gas.
- May experience "the shakes."
- May be hot or cold.

Comfort measures

- Rest between contractions.
- Continue to use the comfort measures that have been working for you.
- This is the shortest but most intense stage and you will be ready to push soon.
- Rely on your support person as much as you need to.
- Use breathing techniques if you have the urge to push before your cervix is completely dilated.

Role of support person

- Remember that the birth is near and offer encouraging words.
- Realize that you may have difficulty helping during this phase.
- Remain together; reduce distractions (environmental or family).
- Maintain eye contact and use short, simple statements.
- Support breathing and stay focused.
- Work in a calm, organized manner.
- Remember, this phase may be difficult for both of you.

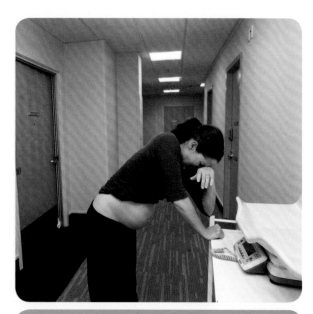

Transition in a snapshot:

- Cervix dilates from 8 to 10 cm.
- Contractions range from 1 ½ to 2 minutes apart.
- Contractions last between 60 to 90 seconds in duration, are intense and can double peak.
- Phase can last for a few minutes to 3 hours.
- Your baby begins to rotate toward your backbone with their chin tucked on their chest.

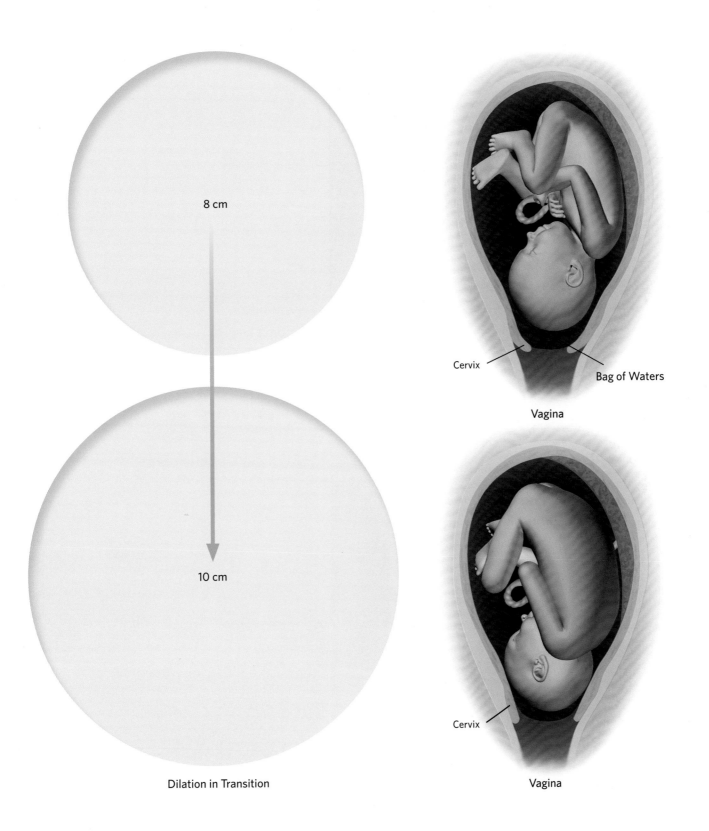

8 cm

10 cm

Dilation in Transition

Cervix

Bag of Waters

Vagina

Cervix

Vagina

Second Stage of Labor

The technique for pushing is a natural one. You will feel the natural urge to push as your baby's head moves through the birth canal. Your goal is to consciously keep your pelvic floor muscles relaxed and respond to the natural urge to push. The natural urges will have you pushing for about 5 to 7 seconds at a time about 3 to 4 times during one contraction. Following the natural urge to push can decrease your fatigue, prevent *perineal* trauma and delay your active pushing time.

Pushing (See page 40-41 for positions)

Emotions and reactions

- Finds strength and energy; a "light at the end of the tunnel" feeling.
- May find it difficult to push in the beginning; learn how "on-the-job" since there is no practicing.
- May find pushing is a relief — can now participate with the work of the contractions.
- Occasionally belch, pass gas or stool.
- May continue with the shakes.
- May experience a burning and stretching sensation as baby moves down the birth canal.

Physical changes

- May have contractions less frequently; they may space out to be every 2 to 5 minutes, lasting 45 to 90 seconds long.
- May have a natural urge to bear down with contractions like having a bowel movement.
- May see or feel bulging of the *perineum* and rectum along with the bloody vaginal show.
- May fall asleep between contractions.
- May make noises or grunt between contractions due to the enormous amount of pressure felt.
- May have natural rest period before there is an urge to push. Take this time to rest and relax.
- If you do not feel a strong urge to push, changing positions, like squatting, can help.

Comfort measures

- Rest between contractions.
- Continue to use any comfort measures that have been working for you.
- Rely on your support person as much as you need.
- Focus on the imminent arrival of your baby.

Role of support person

- Offer verbal encouragement every step of the way.
- Give physical support for the pushing positions chosen.
- Offer a cool washcloth and ice chips.
- May need to help them pant/blow as the head crowns, if healthcare provider requests to slow or stop pushing.
- Have staff help you with "crowd control" if it becomes a problem; focus your full attention on the birth of your baby.

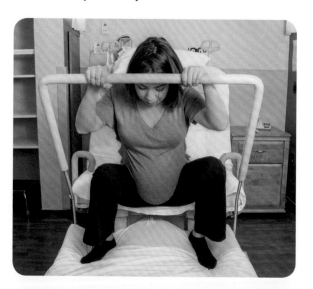

Second stage in a snapshot:

- Cervix is completely dilated to birth of baby.
- Contractions range from 2 to 5 minutes apart.
- Contractions last from 45 to 90 seconds.
- This stage can last from one contraction to 3 hours on average.

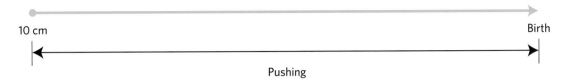

10 cm

Birth

Pushing

Pushing

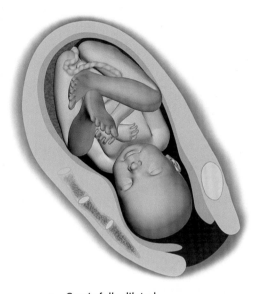

- Cervix fully dilated.
- Baby begins rotating toward your back.
- Baby's chin tucked on their chest.

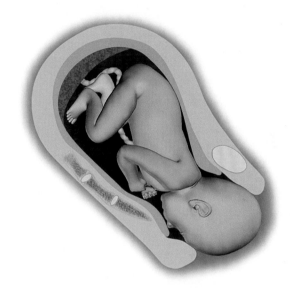

- Baby's head appears at vagina — called *crowning*.

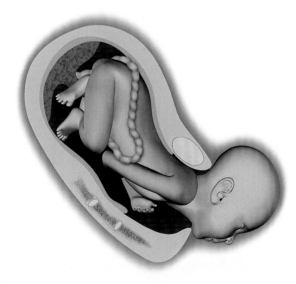

- Head is out and facing the floor. Extension of the baby's head.

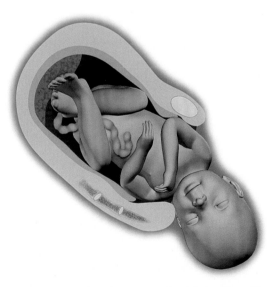

- Head rotates to the side to align with shoulders — called *restitution*.

Pushing Positions

Side-lying

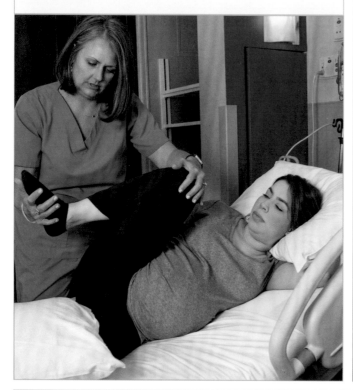

Upright

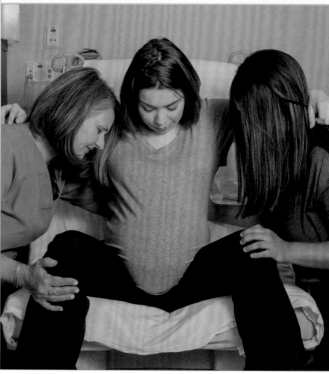

Tug of War

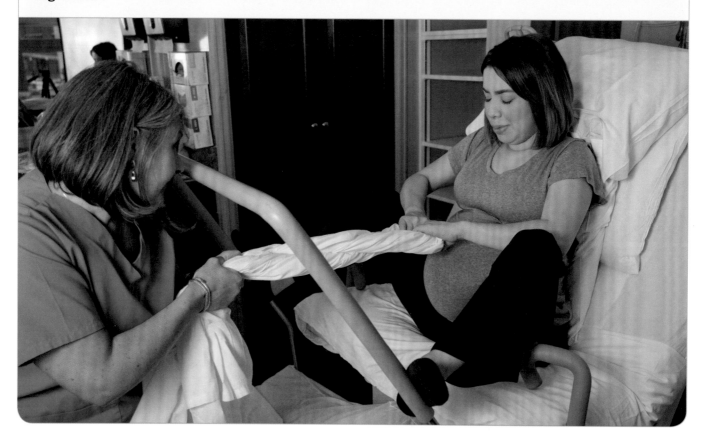

Squat Bar

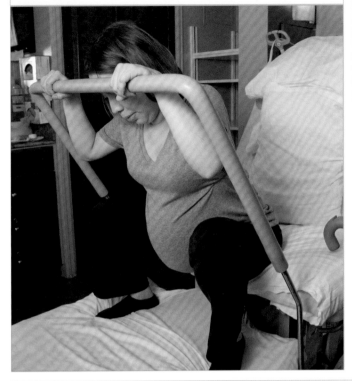

Rebozo Squat

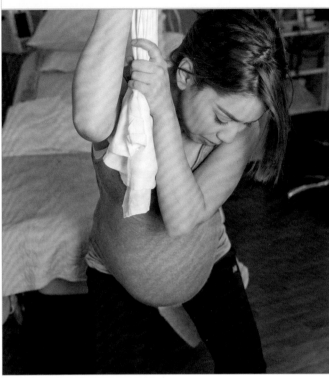

Hands and Knees

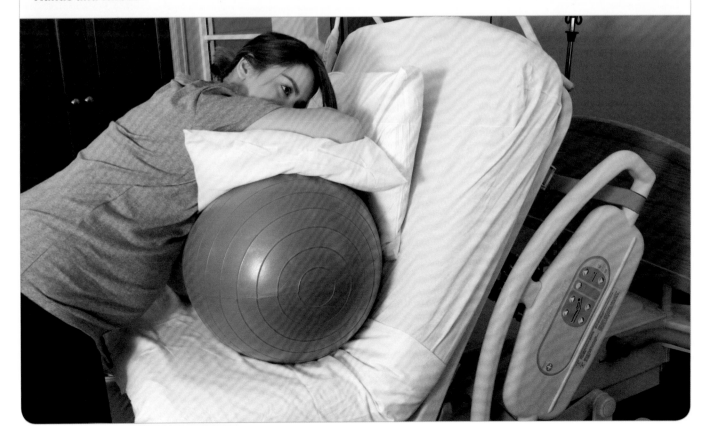

Third Stage of Labor

After the birth of your baby, the placenta will take a few minutes to separate from the wall of the uterus and be pushed out. The contractions will not be as strong, but you may still need to use relaxation techniques during this process. Your healthcare provider may ask you to give a couple of small pushes to help the placenta come out.

Birth of the Placenta

Emotions and reactions

- May be screaming with delight or may be overwhelmed and want to sleep.
- Involved with how the baby is doing; asking questions about the baby's well-being.
- A sense of relief!

Physical changes

- Slowing of contractions after birth of the baby.
- Shrinking of uterus to grapefruit size; now found at the level of the belly button.
- May feel cold, shaky and sick to your stomach.

Comfort measures

- Use relaxation techniques during the delivery of the placenta.
- Focus on your new baby!
- Use a warm blanket with your baby placed skin-to-skin if you're feeling cold or shaky.

Role of the support person

- Enjoy your new baby!
- Continue to support their physical and emotional needs.
- Offer words of congratulations for a job well done!

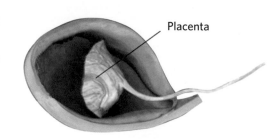

Third stage in a snapshot:
- This stage begins when the baby is born and ends with the delivery of the placenta.
- The birth of the placenta can take anywhere from 5 minutes to 1 hour.
- Remind healthcare professionals if you are planning on keeping your placenta.
- You may need to sign a release form from the hospital to do so.
- Arrange for the placenta to be picked up promptly.

What Happens to My Placenta After Birth?

What happens to your placenta after it is expelled depends on several factors. The placenta can give the healthcare provider insight into different aspects of your pregnancy and birth process. With this in mind, your healthcare provider may elect to have the placenta sent to pathology for further inspection. If your healthcare provider does not deem this necessary, there are two more options for the placenta. It can be discarded, or it can be taken home with you. You may need to sign a release form in order to take your placenta. Please note that if you are planning on taking your placenta home with you, you will need to arrange for it to be picked up promptly due to its need for refrigeration. Most birthing venues do not provide that service.

Placenta

 Find supporting tools and videos in YoMingo.

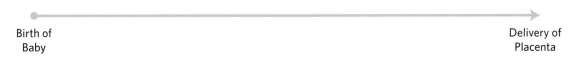

Birth of
Baby

Delivery of
Placenta

Birth of the Placenta

Cutting the Umbilical Cord

Cutting the umbilical cord is one of the final steps in the labor process. The cord that has transported vital nutrients and energy to the growing baby, while also eliminating waste, can now be severed. The cord will be clamped with a small plastic device near the base of the umbilical cord on the baby. A second clamp will define the area where the cord can be cut with a pair of scissors. The umbilical cord does not contain any nerve fibers so it can be cut painlessly. As to who will cut the cord — that decision is up to you!

Delayed Cord Clamping

Expanding evidence supports this practice, which is becoming common in many birth venues. With delayed cord clamping, the cutting of the cord will not occur until the flow of blood from the placenta to the baby has stopped or the placenta has been delivered. This may take about 1 to 5 minutes or longer. The benefit of delayed cord clamping is the increased blood volume received by the baby from the placenta. This blood is rich in iron, which adds to the baby's own iron stores to promote healthy brain development.

Cord Blood Banking

- Stem cells are unique in that they have the potential to treat numerous diseases and disorders.
- These cells are found in the umbilical cord where they can be collected following birth.
- The collected blood containing the stem cells can then be stored for future use if needed.
- There are private and public cord blood banks in the U.S.
- Cost of storage varies depending on the private bank chosen for storage.

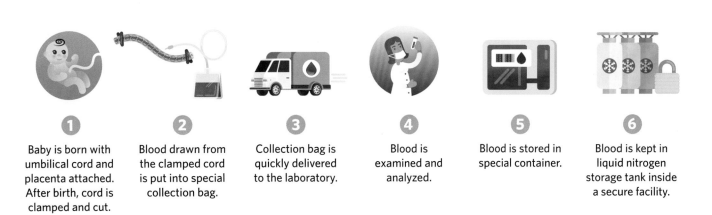

1. Baby is born with umbilical cord and placenta attached. After birth, cord is clamped and cut.
2. Blood drawn from the clamped cord is put into special collection bag.
3. Collection bag is quickly delivered to the laboratory.
4. Blood is examined and analyzed.
5. Blood is stored in special container.
6. Blood is kept in liquid nitrogen storage tank inside a secure facility.

Recovery Care

During this period your blood pressure, heart rate and temperature will be monitored closely for the first hour. The top of your uterus, known as the fundus, is now found around your belly button. Your healthcare provider will check it by using their hands to feel for the top of your uterus. It is important that the uterus remains firm. If not, there could be excessive vaginal bleeding. Your healthcare provider will massage your fundus frequently to keep it contracted and prevent bleeding. This can be uncomfortable. Sometimes more medication is given to keep the uterus firm. Breastfeeding and skin-to-skin contact with your baby also help the uterus to contract and minimize bleeding.

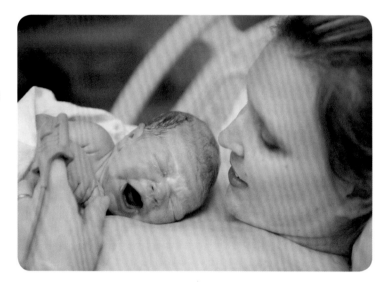

Water Birth

A growing number of people are choosing to give birth while immersed in water. Hydrotherapy, which has many benefits, can be used during the stages of labor and, for some, during the actual birth process. Water birth ideally takes place in a large tub that is comfortable and deep enough for the water to cover your belly. While this practice is prevalent in home births and birthing centers, water births are also occurring in hospital settings, most often overseen by hospital-based midwifery groups. Birth centers and hospitals have policies, procedures and equipment necessary for water birth. If you wish to have a water birth, please discuss this with your healthcare provider early in your pregnancy.

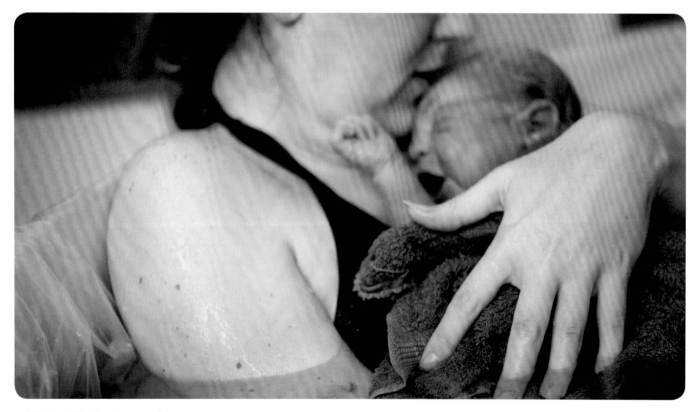

Find supporting tools and videos in YoMingo.

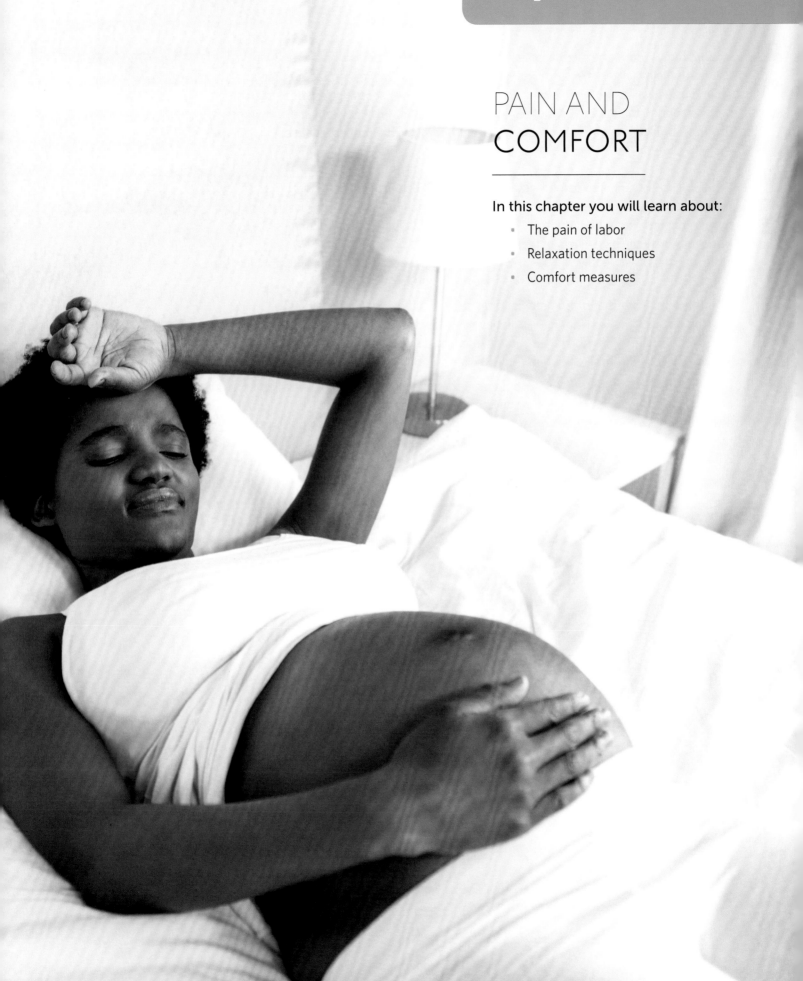

Chapter 4

PAIN AND COMFORT

In this chapter you will learn about:

- The pain of labor
- Relaxation techniques
- Comfort measures

The Pain of Labor

Undoubtedly, one of the most pressing concerns a pregnant person has is the pain that will be experienced during childbirth. Pain is a very personal and subjective experience. We learn about pain and our reaction to it from those around us as well as from our own individual experiences. Becoming knowledgeable about the birth process will help you understand the causes of pain during labor. With this knowledge, and in light of your own perception of pain, you will learn constructive ways to navigate through the process of labor.

How Does the Body Respond to Pain?

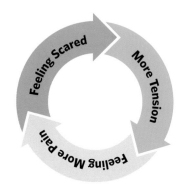

When facing a suspected painful situation, our usual response is one of fear. People don't typically want to feel pain. Foreseeing a painful stimulus causes tension to build in our bodies. So when the fearfully anticipated pain occurs, it is magnified by the high levels of tension that have built up. Due to the elevated levels of pain, most people will be even more fearful of subsequent pain. And so the cycle begins again. This is known as the Fear-Tension-Pain Cycle.

What this means is that if you enter labor already afraid of what you will feel — that the pain will be excruciating — you have already set yourself up to enter the fear-tension-pain cycle. And when you feel the first pangs of labor, your fears will be realized as your already tense body will experience the pain to its fullest.

Unfortunately, there are further consequences to the fear-tension-pain cycle. Not only is there the increase in physical pain, but, in the face of fear, the body releases chemicals that divert the major supply of blood in your body away from "non-essential organs." This blood is then redirected to your limbs so that you can escape the situation that has caused you fear. In the world of labor, this means that if you are afraid, your uterus, a nonessential organ, will be left with little to no blood supply to fuel the contractions to accomplish their purpose. Your labor will slow until the perceived threat is gone.

How do I break or stay away from this cycle?

* Knowledge of the process of labor.
* A positive attitude.
* An understanding of the importance of relaxation.

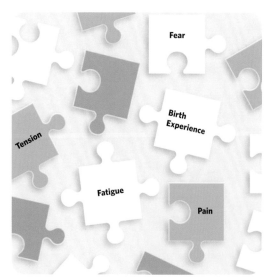

The birth experience can be like a puzzle — fragmented pieces which leave you unsure how they fit together.

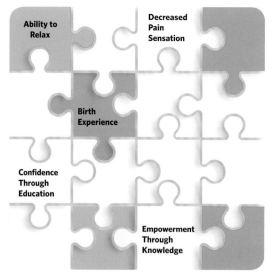

Education and knowledge of the birth process will set up a positive responsive pattern and a positive experience.

46

Where Does the Pain Come From?

Physical

- The thinning out and dilation of the cervix.
- The pressure of your baby's head during the descent down your birth canal.
- Lactic acid build-up as the uterus contracts.
- The contracting uterus putting pressure on the bladder, rectum and pelvis.
- The size and position of your baby.
- The opening of the vagina and perineum.

Due to the wide range of the different sources of pain associated with labor and birth, it would be wise for you to become familiar with the many coping techniques available in order to navigate through this process. Before listing the specific coping strategies, it is important for you to know why the following techniques are effective in diminishing the pain during labor and birth.

Mental

- Your personal beliefs and cultural conditioning in response to pain.
- The quality of support that you have during labor and birth.
- Your mental well-being prior to labor and birth.

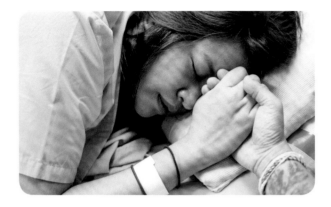

How Does the Body Feel Pain?

In order to understand how certain coping strategies can block pain, it is important for you to know how the body processes pain. There are both anatomic and physiologic mechanisms by which the body transmits painful and soothing stimuli to the brain which results in what you physically feel. Broken down, what this means is that different sensations are delivered to the brain for interpretation along two nerve pathways. The larger nerve pathway delivers soothing sensations, stemming from the skin layer to the brain such as touch, heat, cold, scents, sounds and pressure. This nerve pathway carries these sensations very quickly to the brain. The smaller nerve pathway delivers stimuli such as burning, aching, and sharp pains. This is a slow-moving pathway.

The brain will only interpret one pathway at a time, and while both pathways are delivering sensations and messages to the brain, the faster, larger pathway will receive priority over the slower, smaller nerve pathway. Eventually, the painful stimuli may break through, at which time you will need to change your soothing sensation.

What does this mean? When a painful stimuli is experienced, if a pleasurable sensation occurs at the same time, the pleasurable sensation will reach the brain first, lessening the impact of the painful stimuli. This is called the *Gate Control Theory* and this is what will enable you to progress through labor with understanding instead of fear. Your body already has the framework. Let's discuss how to use it!

2 Nerve Pathways   **Brain**

The smaller nerve pathway delivers sharp pains and is a slow-moving pathway.

The larger nerve pathway, which is a fast-moving pathway, delivers soothing sensations stemming from the skin such as touch, heat, cold, scents, sounds and pressure.

Find supporting tools and videos in YoMingo.

Comfort Measures in Labor

Comfort measures can help you manage the discomforts of labor. This section will help you to understand several techniques that are useful in providing natural pain relief. They can be very effective during the different phases and stages of your labor and birth. Be sure to practice them in class and at home with your labor partner.

Relaxation

Relaxation is an active, purposeful activity in which you consciously release tension. Relaxing your muscles helps to reduce physical tension and pain. It also provides a feeling of emotional well-being which reduces anxiety and, in turn, reduces your sensitivity to pain. Relaxation and rhythmic breathing techniques used during labor help to enhance the progress of your labor and relieve pain. These techniques shift your focus away from the sensation of contractions.

Basic Relaxation

How does your body handle stress? In what area of your body do you carry tension? Become aware of your body by systematically reviewing and practicing basic relaxation techniques with your partner. Knowing the difference between tension and relaxation will help you develop a better sense of awareness that is critical as you prepare for your journey through labor.

Progressive Relaxation

After learning body awareness, progressive relaxation helps you to understand the feeling of tension. Your labor partner will cue you to tense and relax different muscle groups from head to toe. As you tense a certain muscle group, be conscious of the feeling of tension. Try to keep the rest of your body relaxed. Then relax the muscle group that is tense and notice the difference.

Touch Relaxation

A great tool in developing your relaxation skills and working as a team with your labor partner is touch relaxation. Your partner will tell you a muscle group to tense. When you feel your partner's touch, relax that area. If practiced faithfully together, this will be a nonverbal cue, through your labor partner's touch, to relax an area of your body that your partner thinks is tense. You and your partner may have worked together to perfect other relaxation skills. That is great! The most important thing is working as a team.

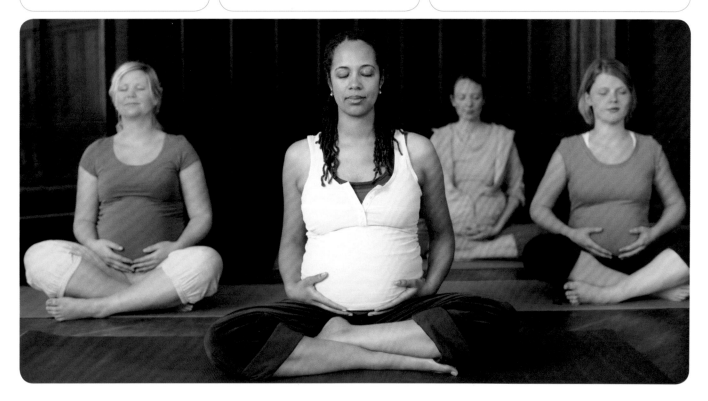

Breathing Patterns

There is no magic to breathing. During labor, however, the use of different breathing techniques will allow you to take your mind off your discomfort and to focus on something else. Our brains will only perceive what we are concentrating on. Everything else is a distraction. You can consciously choose to make yourself think about your breathing instead of the discomfort from the contractions. Breathing techniques also help you remember to not hold your breath during a contraction.

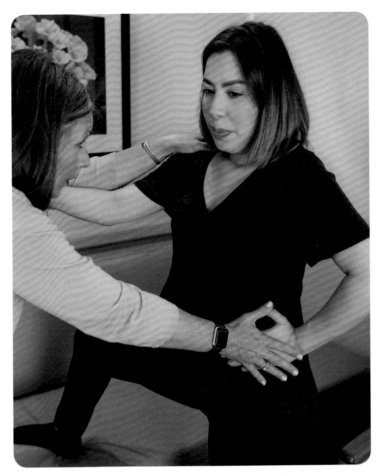

There is no right or wrong way to breathe. Your breathing style will be your own — whatever feels appropriate to you at that time in your labor. There are no special rules for how many breaths per minute, whether to breathe through the mouth or nose, or whether to make sounds or not. The key to breathing is to purposefully focus on air coming into your body and the air leaving your body. You will receive the most benefits from breathing techniques if you use two common components: a cleansing breath and a focal point. For some, a description of different breathing patterns is helpful. Here are three such techniques that can be practiced and personalized.

Slow Breathing

This is a relaxed and comfortable breathing pattern. Some patients find that slow breathing works well during early labor. Breathe in slowly and deeply. With each slow breath out, relax your face, shoulders, arms, and working your way towards your toes. Keeping your body as relaxed as possible is important because it is a basic way to help relieve pain and tension.

Light, Quick Breathing

Some people find that light, quick breathing works well when contractions become stronger and last longer. At the beginning of the contraction, take a deep cleansing breath. Continue with slow breathing in and out. As the contraction increases in intensity, use shallow, rhythmical breaths in and out. As each contraction eases, end with another deep cleansing breath.

Pant-Pant Blow Breathing

Pant-pant blow can be helpful if you have the strong urge to bear down and push, but your cervix has not fully dilated. Take a deep breath in. Breathe out with short pants and then a longer breath. Pant-pant blow. Repeat until the contraction eases and end with a deep cleansing breath.

Hands-On Relief

Using a hands-on approach for pain relief does not require fancy techniques. Touch can convey pain-reducing messages by sending sensations of pleasure to the receptors in the brain. People vary on the types of touch that they enjoy or find helpful. Some find gentle pressure irritating while in labor, but it might be ideal for someone else.

Touch and Massage

Touch and massage have been proven to be very healing in general and very beneficial in reducing pain sensations during labor. Touch soothes the body through simple hand-holding and gentle stroking of the arms, legs or abdomen. In labor, your body naturally releases endorphins that are "morphine-like." These pain-relieving chemicals give a sense of well-being. With massage and touch, more endorphins can be released as long as you stay as relaxed as possible. Tension and stress tend to cancel out the endorphins with hormones called catecholamines. They are released when you are under stress and cause the "fight or flight" response. These hormones make your heart beat faster, your breathing more rapid, and your muscles more tense. During labor, you want all the morphine-like chemicals you can get!

Effleurage

Effleurage is a type of massage using light pressure applied over a wide area of the body. Light effleurage promotes relaxation, alleviates pain and encourages sleep. Perform it in a circular motion with the hands relaxed and palms on the body. Always keep the momentum on the upward stroke, easing the pressure on the return movement. Use a flat-hand stroke on the arms, legs and broad flat surface of the back.

Effleurage with only the fingertips gliding (rather than the whole hand) is called feathering. Some people enjoy using feathering over their abdomen during contractions. Effleurage can also be done with a cupped-hand on areas that are sensitive, such as the calf muscles.

Pressure

Applying pressure to certain areas of the body has been proven to decrease stress, tension and painful sensations. A good example is a headache. Without realizing it, you may have applied pressure to your temples with your fingertips and, while moving them in a circular motion, you notice that your head is actually feeling better. You have just put the gate control theory to practice! Pressure often helps reduce the pain of *back labor*.

Double Hip Squeeze

The double hip squeeze is a type of pressure applied to the hips that can relieve lower back pain. During labor, the pressure of the baby's head stretches the pelvis. The hip squeeze pushes the pelvis back into a relaxed position which relieves the pressure of the stretch. Your partner, doula or other support person can gently place their palms on your hip bones to find the proper placement. Keeping one hand on each hip bone and thumbs pointed toward the spine forming a "W", they can push the hip bones "in and up" toward the body. You can be standing or leaning over the bed or a birthing ball. Swaying gently during the contraction as they squeeze may help ease the pain. The hip squeeze can be varied with counter pressure on the lower back. This can be hard work for the support person over time. They will probably need a break, so make sure that you have a backup person available.

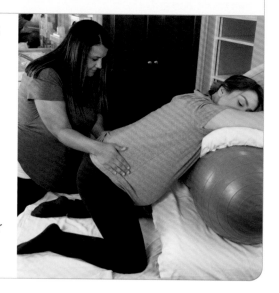

Focus

You will use your mental energy to focus on the birth of your baby. Try some of these options to help you focus your mind. You may also want to try a mantra, where you repeat a word or short phrase. The one that is right is the one that works for you. *Meditation* is an effective way to reduce anxiety and stress and produce endorphins, the pleasure hormone. Practicing meditation during pregnancy is helpful since the effects of meditation actually improve with time.

Cleansing Breath

At the beginning and end of each contraction, take a deep, exaggerated breath in through your nose and out through your mouth. This deep breath will give both you and your baby an extra boost of oxygen and signal you to relax and focus. It will also serve as a cue to your partner that a contraction has begun. The cleansing breath serves as a release for you and a reminder to relax between contractions.

Focal Point

Focusing all your attention on one thing allows distracting thoughts and images to simply pass by. Any point of focus can work — a word or sound, a phrase, a photograph or a meaningful object. Meditation is also an effective way of shutting out other concerns. Add an item to your labor bag that you feel will help you to focus.

Guided Imagery

The technique of visualization, or using your imagination, does not work for everyone but could be of great assistance to you. Using visualization or guided imagery involves focusing on a mental image — a place in your mind that is special to you. Use your senses — smell the scents, see the colors and hear the sounds. Share your special place with your labor support person, and they may be able to walk you through the technique.

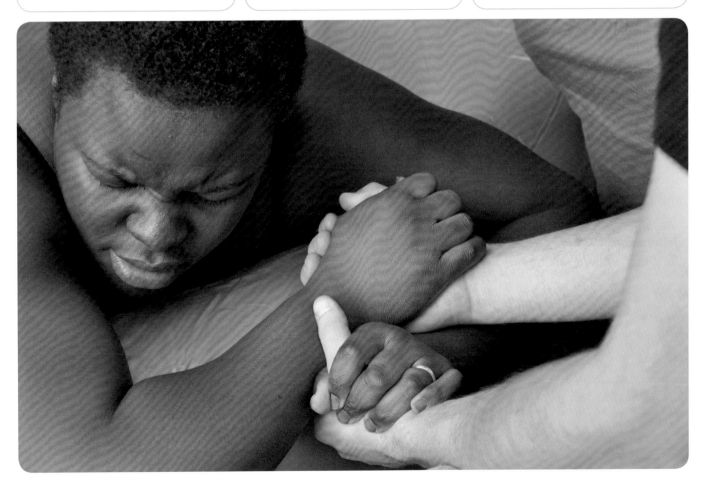

Environmental Influences

It can be easy to dismiss the effectiveness of adjusting the lighting in a room or even the temperature. Please communicate to your labor partner how you are best able to relax. Do you like a bright room or do you prefer for the lights to be dimmed? How about the temperature — do you like it to be cooler or do you find it easier to relax when the room is warm? These are relatively simple changes to make but they can ultimately make a significant difference in your ability to relax during labor.

Aromatherapy

Aromatherapy, which is an ancient art form, is the use of essential oils of plants and herbs. It is a safe, non-invasive, natural treatment for both the body and mind. Many birth professionals and midwives are now adding aromatherapy into their practice as a gentle and effective way of helping relax the laboring person, ease pain and calm anxiety. Even if you choose conventional methods of pain relief, aromatherapy can calm your mind, fortify your mood, soothe pain and alleviate discomfort.

Benefits of aromatherapy during labor include:

- Certain oils help energize and strengthen, giving you the confidence to approach labor with a bit more calm.
- Can be used by your labor partner for massage and can help alleviate the pain of contractions, control nerves and ease anxiety.
- Can be used in a soothing bath.
- Some oils may relieve nausea.
- In transition, when it is common to feel tired and discouraged, essentials oils can be used to lift mood and ease fatigue.

Talk to your healthcare provider, midwife or doula for recommendations on which essential oils are best to use during labor.

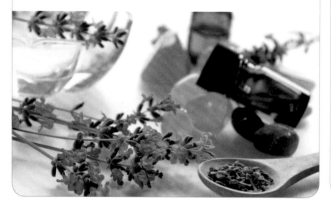

Heat and Cold

Warmth is extremely effective in reducing pain and creating relaxation. Warm water, a hot water bottle, a heating pad or warm compresses to your lower back can all be effective. Cold compresses or ice bags can also be helpful for pain relief. Try alternating heat and cold or use heat and cold on separate parts of your body at the same time. Change your heat and cold locations about every twenty minutes to give you the most relief.

Music

Music envelops you and helps you relax by drowning out any distractions taking place around you. It also helps to soothe your environment. Select music that is comforting to you. Whatever you choose to use when practicing your relaxation techniques, bring along with you to the hospital. You will find it to be more effective using music you enjoy.

Hydrotherapy

Hydrotherapy is the use of water to provide safe effective non-pharmacological pain relief. It has both physical and psychological benefits. Immersion hydrotherapy puts you in a tub with water deep enough to cover your belly. You can also use water therapy by sitting or standing in a shower. Keep the water temperature about 98-100°F and use caution if you become dizzy or lightheaded. Fetal monitoring can be done intermittently or with a mobile device.

Benefits of hydrotherapy:

- Safe.
- Effective.
- Provides comfort.
- Produces relaxation.
- Easy to move around.

Labor Position Aids

There are items you can use to aid you with position changes, which can be a simple way to help relieve pain. During labor your baby is making tiny movements that are very important to the birthing process. Using different positions while in labor will assist your baby in making these movements.

Birthing Ball

Using a birthing ball can help you into different upright positions and help you to labor effectively. It may even shorten your labor by about an hour and help reduce the pain of contractions. Some midwives recommend a birthing ball to help cope at home in early labor. You may find you instinctively sway and rock in rhythm with your contractions. A birthing ball gives great support while you do this.

Ways to use your birthing ball during labor include:

- Sit astride the ball and rock your pelvis from side to side or back and forth.

- Lean on your birthing ball from a kneeling position on the floor.

- Get into a hands-and-knees position by hugging your ball and lift your bottom up from a kneeling position. You can then rock your pelvis from side to side.

- Lean over your ball from a standing position, with the ball on the bed or another surface.

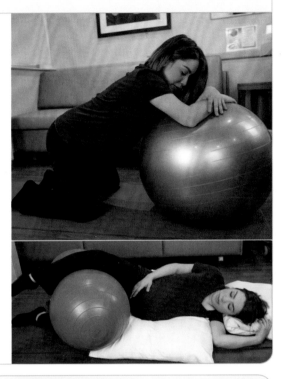

Rebozo

A rebozo is a shawl, typically made out of handwoven fabric, whose use has been adapted to benefit people both before and during labor. Before labor, the rebozo can be used to aid in the correct positioning of the baby with a technique called "sifting." To do this, the shawl is positioned on a soft surface with the pregnant person laying in the center of the shawl in a perpendicular direction. The labor support person then gathers the long ends of the rebozo from both sides and gently "jiggles" them. This same technique can be used if they get on all fours with the rebozo positioned to cradle their pregnant abdomen.

During labor, the rebozo can be suspended from the ceiling or doorframe to assist the laboring person in a supported squat. They can put the rebozo underneath their arms like a sling to support some of their weight or hold the ends of the suspended rebozo with both hands and pull on it as they squat down. When it is time, pushing efforts can be enhanced by using a "tug-of-war" technique on the rebozo – either with the support person or by looping the rebozo over a squat bar.

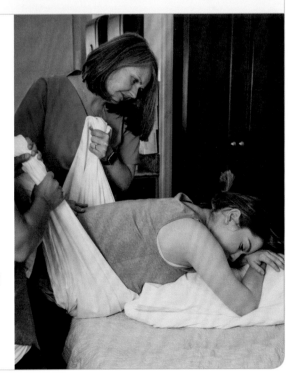

Changing Positions

Staying in one position during labor can increase tension in the body, while moving regularly can significantly reduce pain. Moving while remaining in an upright position is beneficial to both the progress of labor and to your comfort level. Some examples of position changes that allow your body to take advantage of gravity and movement and also encourage the repositioning and downward movement of the baby are: walking, rocking, standing, swaying and slow dancing.

Walking/Standing

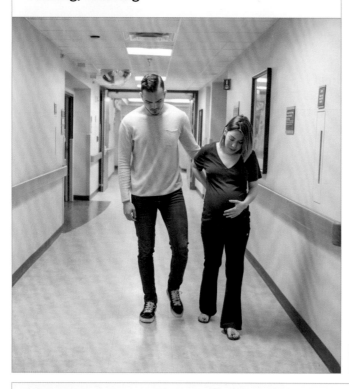

Squatting

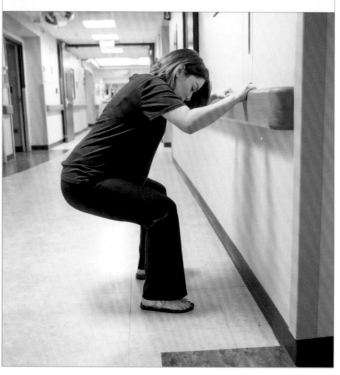

Side-Lying

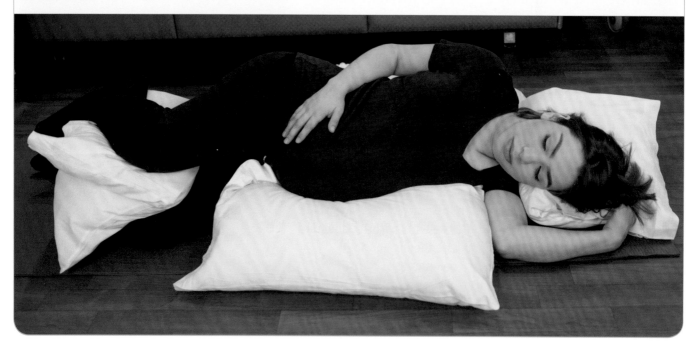

Kneeling on Hands and Knees

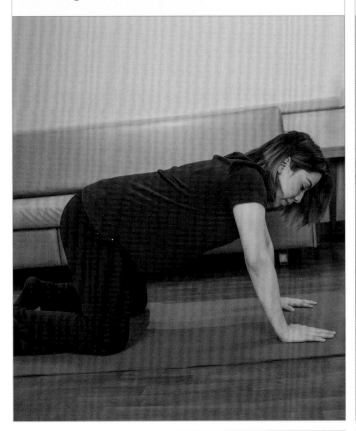

Lunging

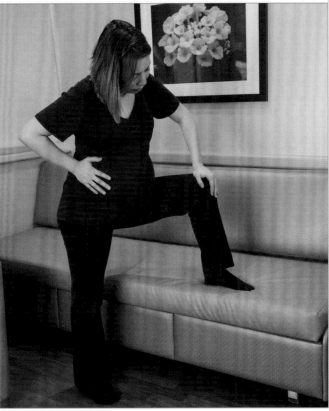

Sitting

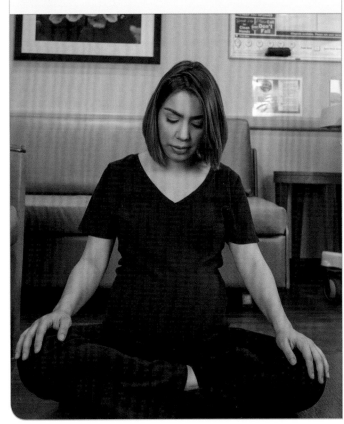

Slow Dancing

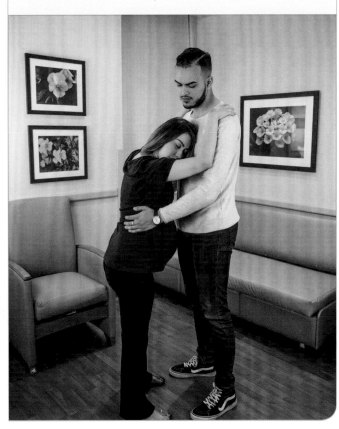

Back Labor

Not everyone has back labor. The pain of back labor may be intense and interfere with the ability to relax. This situation is generally caused by the baby's face facing upward, or occiput posterior, causing more pressure on the pelvis and tailbone. This pressure comes from the hard part of the baby's head pressing on the pelvic bones. Changing positions frequently can help to rotate the baby's head. Having the baby's face pointing toward your back (occiput anterior) is more favorable for birth. Forward-leaning positions are effective in promoting the rotation of the baby as well as allowing free access for your labor partner to use counterpressure on your lower back.

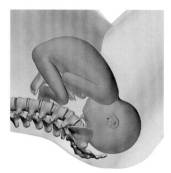 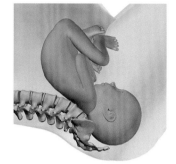 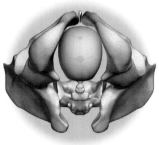 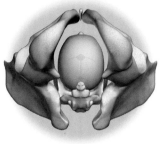

Head is in anterior position (Occiput Anterior or OA)   Head is in posterior position (Occiput Posterior or OP)

To apply counterpressure, have your labor partner press firmly against the small of your lower back with a closed fist or the heel of their hand. You will tell them exactly where to apply pressure and how hard to push. This pressure technique helps tremendously in reducing the discomfort associated with back labor. The use of cold temperatures (such as an ice pack) or warmth (such as a heating pad) can be used as alternatives to counterpressure or in conjunction with it.

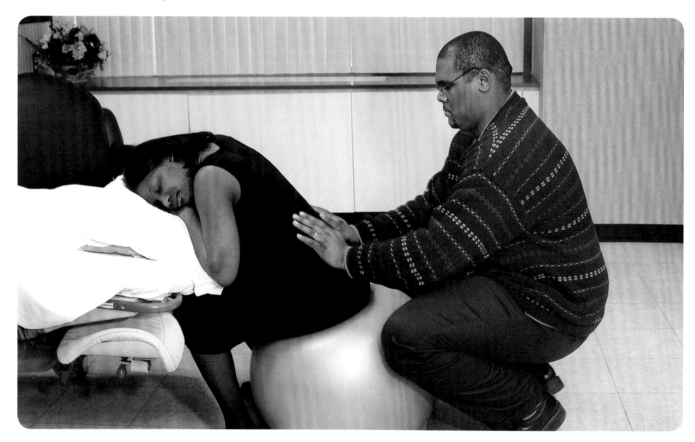

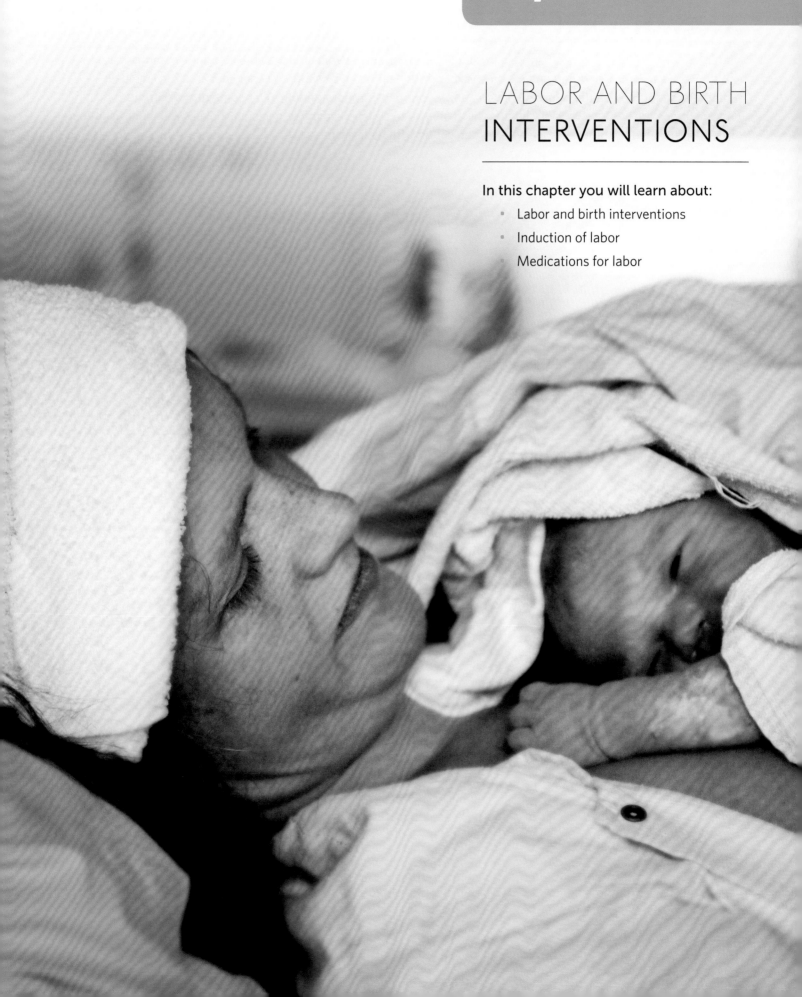

Chapter 5

LABOR AND BIRTH
INTERVENTIONS

In this chapter you will learn about:

- Labor and birth interventions
- Induction of labor
- Medications for labor

Labor and Birth Interventions

Interventions can play an important role in your labor experience. While you may be planning an unmedicated birth with as few medical interventions as possible, your healthcare provider may suggest an unexpected intervention for the health and safety of you and/or your baby. Understanding what some of the common interventions are before your labor begins will allow you to be involved in the decision-making with your healthcare provider. Asking questions and openly communicating with your birth team will guide your care and help to provide a satisfactory birth experience for you.

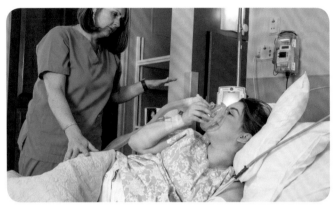 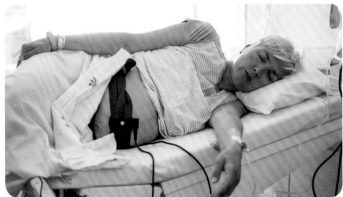

Intravenous Fluids

Intravenous therapy, called an IV, may or may not be part of your routine care depending on where you plan to give birth. The need for IV fluids should be discussed with your healthcare provider before your labor begins.

You may need an IV for medical reasons:

- To treat *Group Beta Strep*.
    - A bacteria found in the vaginal canal that is harmless to you but can cause serious respiratory complications in your baby.
    - Is tested for by vaginal swab in the healthcare provider's office during third trimester.
    - If you test positive, you will receive antibiotics during labor in order to eliminate the GBS bacteria.
- For intravenous antibiotic therapy.
- To treat fever during prolonged labor.
- To protect against disease or infection during a cesarean birth.

If you choose to have an epidural, it is a requirement for you to receive intravenous fluids.

Advantages	Disadvantages	Alternative
<ul><li>A "safety net" in case of an emergency.</li><li>Keeps you hydrated which can help labor progress.</li><li>Required for epidural or other medical interventions such as medication administration.</li></ul>	<ul><li>Discomfort at IV site.</li><li>IV makes it difficult to move around freely for comfort measures.</li></ul>	<ul><li>A saline lock or venous access port can be placed and used only when necessary.</li><li>This may be a good compromise if you do not wish to have a continuous IV during labor.</li><li>Share your thoughts with your healthcare provider to ensure you are both in agreement prior to labor.</li></ul>

Induced Labor

Induction of labor can be done several ways if labor has not started naturally. The method will depend on your reason for induction and your healthcare provider's decisions. Induction is generally reserved for those pregnancies with certain medical problems or other special circumstances.

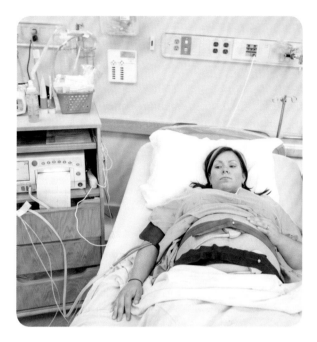

Medical reasons for inducing labor may include:

- High blood pressure.
- Diabetes.
- Rh disease.
- Overdue pregnancy.
- Small-for-dates pregnancy.
- Ruptured membranes.
- Known complications with the fetus.

Ripening of the Cervix

Normally, prostaglandins produced during pregnancy will painlessly start the ripening process (shortening, softening and dilating the cervix) during the last weeks of pregnancy. If your healthcare provider feels that an induction is necessary and the cervix is not ripe, they may choose to start your induction by ripening your cervix. You may receive a medicated suppository that is placed in the vagina next to the cervix. These suppositories contain prostaglandins and help to prepare the cervix for induction. Another way your healthcare provider may ripen your cervix is by inserting a small silicone tube with a balloon on the end into the cervix. The balloon is then filled with water to physically begin dilating the cervix. It is typical to remain in the hospital for both prostaglandin use as well as a cervical ripening balloon.

Misoprostol is a medication originally used to treat stomach ulcers. It was discovered that it can also produce uterine contractions. One disadvantage of the medication is that if uterine hyperstimulation occurs, it is more difficult to reverse its effects versus other contraction-stimulating drugs. For this reason, use of Misoprostol remains controversial.

Stripping the Membranes

Stripping the membranes is a procedure that your healthcare provider can perform in their office. During a vaginal exam, one finger passes through the cervix, and in a circular motion the amniotic sac is separated from the wall of the uterus. This causes the body to release oxytocin, which causes contractions. This procedure is not always successful and can be quite uncomfortable. Do not be surprised if you see some bloody show afterwards.

Nipple Stimulation

Nipple stimulation can be performed manually or with the use of a breast pump. During stimulation, the brain directs the release of oxytocin, causing contractions. This should only be done under your healthcare provider's guidance.

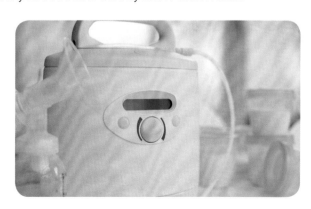

Artificial Rupture of Membranes

Your healthcare provider may artificially rupture your membranes to help labor begin. This is done by inserting an instrument into the cervical canal to rupture the membranes (bag of waters).

Amniotic fluid is generally clear to straw-colored, but may also contain *meconium*, a greenish-brown material which is the baby's first stool. If the fluid is meconium-stained, special attention may be focused on your baby immediately following the birth to prevent lung problems that can result from the baby aspirating (breathing in) the fluid. The amniotic sac has no nerve endings, so this is generally a painless procedure.

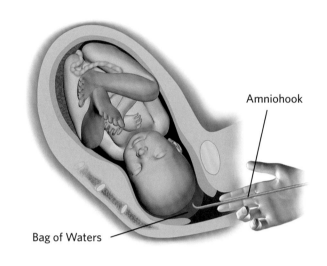

Amniohook

Bag of Waters

Pitocin

Pitocin is a medication used to either start contractions or augment (speed up) labor. This medication is controlled by an intravenous pump set to deliver an amount that stimulates your uterus to contract. It is necessary to receive fetal monitoring if Pitocin is being used.

Concerns:

- Overstimulation of your uterus.
- Infection in you or your baby.
- Increased risk of cesarean birth.
- Uterine rupture.

When Is My Baby Full Term?

According to definitions endorsed by the American Congress of Obstetrics and Gynecologists (ACOG) and the Society for Maternal-Fetal Medicine, a pregnancy is not full term until 39 weeks. This is a change from the old understanding that a pregnancy was considered full term anywhere between 37 weeks and 42 weeks. For many years, people have been told that if they make it to 37 weeks they can assume their babies are ready to be born.

The March of Dimes has been educating the public for some time about elective inductions performed before 39 weeks without a medical reason. This presents a greater risk of health problems for the baby.

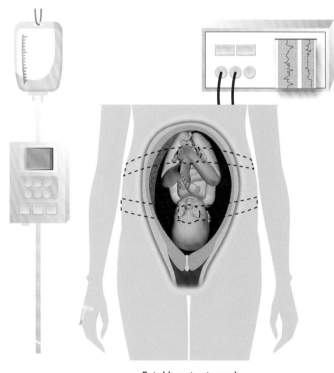

Fetal heart rate and contractions are monitored.

Definitions:

- **Early term:** 37 weeks through 38 weeks and 6 days
- **Full term:** 39 weeks through 40 weeks and 6 days
- **Late term:** 41 weeks through 41 weeks and 6 days
- **Postterm:** 42 weeks and beyond

Assisted Birth

Episiotomy

An *episiotomy* is a surgical incision between the vagina and anus to widen the vaginal opening. This allows more room for the birth of a baby or the use of *forceps*. A local anesthetic is given to avoid discomfort during the episiotomy and repair. Talk to your healthcare provider during your pregnancy about the procedure and any concerns that you may have.

Midline Episiotomy

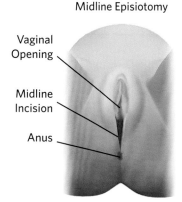

Vaginal Opening

Midline Incision

Anus

Mediolateral Episiotomy

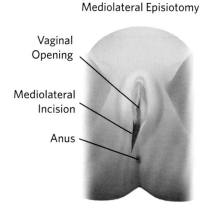

Vaginal Opening

Mediolateral Incision

Anus

Perineal Repair

If your baby needed more room for birth than was allowed by your perineum, and a tear, laceration or episiotomy occured, your healthcare provider will stitch it back together. Prior to proceeding, your caregiver will provide pain medication to ensure your comfort during the repair. You will probably feel some pulling and tugging but not any sharp pain. The suture that is used will dissolve in your tissues, so it will not need to be removed.

Pericare, or how to take care of your perineum or stitches, will be reviewed with you by your nurse or healthcare provider. An ice pack may be applied to your bottom to help with discomfort and swelling.

Forceps and Vacuum Extractor

Forceps and *vacuum extractors* are instruments that can be used during the second stage of labor to assist birth. Your healthcare provider uses them to guide the baby through the birth canal as you continue to push. Both forceps and the vacuum extractor can be beneficial when there is a medical need.

Common reasons for use:

- Fetal distress in which the baby's head is low enough in the pelvis for the baby to be born more quickly and safely than with a cesarean birth.
- Baby's head has not turned toward your back.
- Inability to push because of *epidural anesthesia*.
- Maternal exhaustion.

Concerns:

- Forceps may cause temporary bruising which tends to fade within 48 hours.
- The suction from the vacuum may cause some swelling of the baby's scalp.
- Increased chance of *jaundice* in babies when vacuum extractors are used.
- May cause injury to the vagina, perineum and anus.

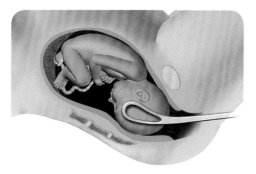

The forceps are gently inserted into the vagina around the baby's head.

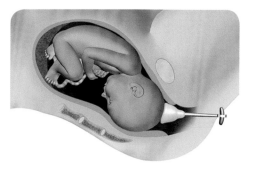

A suction cup is placed on top of the baby's head.

Fetal Monitoring

External Fetal Monitors

An external fetal monitor consists of two devices that are placed on your abdomen once labor begins. One continuously gathers information about the fetal heart rate and the other records the frequency and duration of your uterine contractions.

During labor, your healthcare team will check your baby's heart rate by using a handheld doppler or electronic fetal monitor. The American Congress of Obstetricians and Gynecologists (ACOG) recommends that for healthy, low-risk patients, the baby's heart rate be monitored with a fetal monitor or doppler every 30 minutes in active labor and every 15 minutes during pushing. When risk factors are present, they should be evaluated more frequently or by using *electronic fetal monitoring*.

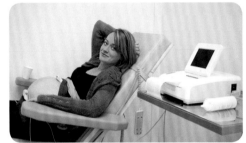

Some health conditions or medications used during labor will require continuous monitoring. You may need continuous monitoring if:

* Your labor is induced or augmented with Pitocin.
* You have an epidural.
* Your baby's heart rate changes.
* You or your baby has a health problem.

Internal Fetal Monitors

When additional information is needed, internal monitors may be used. There are two different devices typically used to obtain more detailed information. The first is called a fetal scalp electrode (FSE). This device is placed on the baby's head and tracks precise fetal heart rate changes. The second instrument is called an intrauterine pressure catheter (IUPC). This device is threaded through the cervix and remains in the uterine cavity next to your baby. The IUPC delivers accurate information about the strength, frequency and duration of contractions.

Internal monitors are not routinely used, and many labors progress smoothly using only external monitors. Only when additional information will help are internal monitors placed. In order to use internal monitors, the amniotic sac must be ruptured and the cervix must be open.

> Telemetry is electronic fetal monitoring without wires. It allows you to have more freedom to get out of bed for comfort strategies such as walking, showering, and using a birthing ball. Telemetry is not available in all hospitals.

Pain Medications

While there are some people who would prefer to labor without using pain medication, there are others who plan to use them. The following is an explanation of the different types of pain medications available, their desired effects on the body, and what the benefits and drawbacks are of each type.

Nirtrous Oxide	**Narcotic Analgesics**	**Local Anesthesia**	**Epidural**	**Spinal Block**	**General Anesthesia**
Inhaled through a mask	Given through IV or injection	Given through injection	Catheter placed in the epidural space	Injected into the subarachnoid space	Given through IV and/or gas

Find supporting tools and videos in YoMingo.

Nitrous Oxide

The use of nitrous oxide is a good choice for those who are undecided about their pain management options as it is non-invasive and simple to use. Nitrous oxide is a gas that you inhale through a face mask during any part of labor. The medication is a mixture of nitrous oxide and oxygen in equal amounts.

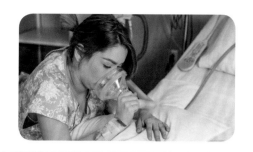

When to Use

- Self-administered by a face mask.
- Can be used during any stage of labor.

Benefits

- Simple to administer and noninvasive.
- Does not interfere with the body's production of oxytocin.
- Does not affect the alertness of your baby.
- Helps with relaxation and decreases the perception of pain.
- Clears your body within five minutes of discontinuation.

Drawbacks

- Not available in all birth facilities.
- Cannot be used after any other type of narcotic or regional anesthetic is used.

Possible Side Effects

- Sedation
- Nausea/vomiting
- Dizziness

Narcotic Analgesics

Examples of these medications, known as opiates, are Demerol, Morphine, Stadol, Nubain, and Fentanyl. This classification of pain medication has a systemic effect which means that the drug will enter the circulatory system and affect the entire body. The medication used will depend upon your healthcare provider and the location you will give birth.

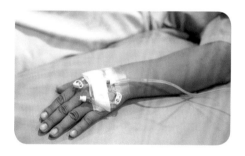

When/How to Use

- In active labor.
- Through IV or injection.

Benefits

- Increases pain tolerance.
- Increases ability to relax.
- Works quickly.
- Does not affect muscles for pushing.
- Does not slow down labor.

Drawbacks

- Does not eliminate pain.
- Can only be administered every so often depending upon the specific medication.
- Only certain times in labor when it can be given.

Possible Side Effects

- May cause nausea, dizziness, drowsiness, disorientation.
- May decrease heart rate, breathing rate or blood pressure.
- Possible allergic reaction.
- Possible temporary breathing problems for your baby.

Local Anesthesia

Local anesthesia is effective for the repair of tears, lacerations or episiotomies after birth. It will affect only the skin area where the medication is given. This anesthesia is often used after an unmedicated birth to provide pain relief if stitches are needed on the perineum.

Epidural Block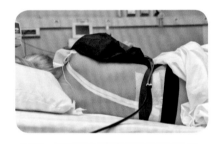

Epidural anesthesia is the most common form of regional anesthesia used during labor. This type of anesthesia will provide pain relief to the lower abdomen during contractions and may even decrease sensation to the legs and birth canal. Receiving epidural anesthesia involves the placement of a small, flexible catheter (tube) in the lower back. Medication is injected into the epidural space which will provide the desired pain relief. Because the length of labor is not known, the epidural catheter will remain securely in place so that you will receive a continuous flow of pain relieving medication until your baby is born.

It is important to understand that in order to receive an epidural, you must first have an IV in place and have good results from your lab tests. After the epidural is in place, you will receive continuous fetal monitoring, frequent blood pressure checks, and possibly a *urinary catheter*. You will also need to remain in the bed due to the numbness of your legs.

Epidural Space

Spinal Space

Points of insertion for spinal and epidural anesthesia.

Possible Side Effects

- **Inadvertent spinal block** — If the membrane that confines the spinal fluid is punctured with the needle or catheter, a higher-than-optimal level of anesthetic may be absorbed. This can also result in a post-spinal headache which may occur following delivery. Sometimes an additional procedure is required to remedy the headache.

- **Blood pressure** — A slight drop in blood pressure is probably one of the most common side effects of epidural blocks. Your blood pressure will be carefully monitored, and you will receive continuous administration of fluids through an IV to minimize this risk.

- **Effect on labor** — Epidural anesthesia can slow labor, especially if it is given too soon. In addition, epidurals may hinder pushing efforts, making the birth of the baby's head more difficult. At other times, it may allow labor to proceed more rapidly than usual.

- **Ineffective pain relief** — The extent of pain relief varies from total relief to no relief at all. Approximately 85% of women get total relief from blocks; others experience only partial relief. Some women have no relief at all.

When not to get an epidural:

There are reasons that may prevent you from being able to get an epidural. If you have or suspect you may have any of the following conditions, you should let your healthcare provider know.

- Bleeding or *coagulation* problems.
- Infection near the site of needle or catheter placement.
- Certain neurological disorders.
- Some types of previous lower back surgery.
- Any significant spinal irregularities.
- A recent tattoo at the injection site.

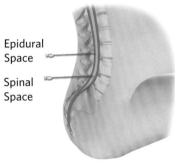 Find supporting tools and videos in YoMingo.

Spinal Block

A spinal block is sometimes referred to as a "spinal." The administration of spinal anesthesia is very similar to that of epidural anesthesia. The main difference is that the anesthetic medication is injected directly into the spinal space (called the subarachnoid space) which provides pain relief for as long as 2 hours. Because spinal medication is typically used for procedures that will last less than 2 hours, there is no need for a catheter to be placed for continuous medication administration. It numbs the lower abdomen, legs and birth canal. It may be the choice of anesthesia for a cesarean birth if an epidural is not already in place.

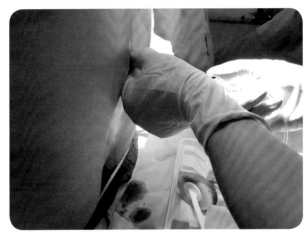

An anesthesiologist or nurse anesthetists will administer an epidural or a spinal block.

General Anesthesia

This type of anesthesia is not administered to a patient who is laboring. It is a systemic anesthetic affecting the whole body including the baby. General anesthesia is used for cesarean births in emergency situations where time is a factor. It is also used for people who need a cesarean and cannot receive an epidural or spinal for the procedure. An anesthesiologist administers the general anesthetic through your IV. You are unconscious and feel no pain after the medication is given. An endotracheal tube is placed down your windpipe and the anesthesiologist "breathes" for you during the procedure. Once the baby is born and the uterus and abdomen incisions are closed, the anesthesiologist reverses the effect of the anesthesia and awakens you. You will likely be groggy for a short time after the procedure. Because regional anesthesia wears off quickly, you will receive immediate pain management assistance in the recovery room.

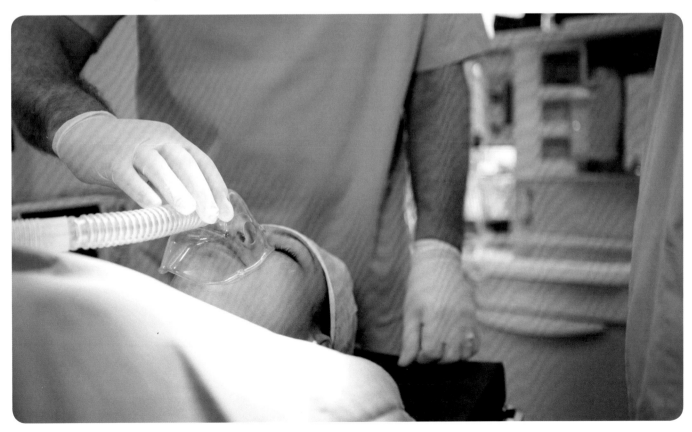

Planning Your Birth

Birth planning encourages you to think through the details of your hopes and preferences for your labor and birth experience. By educating yourself before labor begins, you will better understand your options – especially when it comes to interventions like induction of labor and pain medication. Preparing ahead of time gives you a chance to discuss with both your labor partner and your healthcare provider how you would like your labor and birth handled.

It will help to find out all of the intervention policies and procedures that are considered "routine" in your birthing facility. If you don't agree with a policy or procedure, you should discuss it with your healthcare provider. As you learn more about what to expect during labor and birth, you will likely identify details that you want to include in your plan. An important thing to remember is that everyone has the same goal of a safe labor and birth for you and your baby.

There is no way to predict in advance exactly what may happen during labor or birth, or how a certain intervention may affect you or your baby. Being well-informed and understanding the reason for an intervention will help you make an educated decision if one is suggested. Stay flexible in your preferences in case things don't go according to your plan because your choice will be important to the health and safety of you and your baby.

As you create a birth plan, start with a list of ideas to help you prioritize. If you want minimal interventions, you may want to list alternatives that could be used. You can find birth plan templates online or your birth facility may have one to guide you. You do not have to have a specific form — a piece of paper listing your thoughts and preferences will work, too.

Become informed, get all of your questions answered, and put plans in place in advance that will help you avoid interventions that may be performed more for convenience than due to medical necessity. It is possible for one intervention to quickly lead to the need for more.

Some tips for avoiding unnecessary interventions:

- Choose a healthcare provider and a birthing facility that have low rates of using common interventions.

- Have conversations during your pregnancy with your labor partner and your healthcare provider about common interventions.

- Discuss options for alternatives to common interventions with your healthcare provider.

- Research interventions and understand how one intervention could lead to another one.

- Review the benefits of having a labor support person and investigate the option for a doula.

- Communicate your desires with your healthcare provider, labor partner, doula, and staff at the birthing facility.

Many people continue to feel discomfort even when pain medication is used. Continue to use your comfort measures to help you with relaxation.

Discuss your preferences for pain medication with your healthcare provider before your labor begins. Share any concerns you may have about the effects on you and your baby. Keep an open mind and know your options ahead of time so that you can make an informed decision during labor.

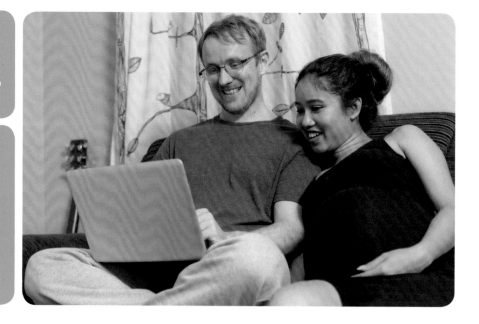

CESAREAN BIRTH

In this chapter you will learn about:

- Reasons for cesarean birth
- Preparation for your baby's birth
- Pain management and recovery

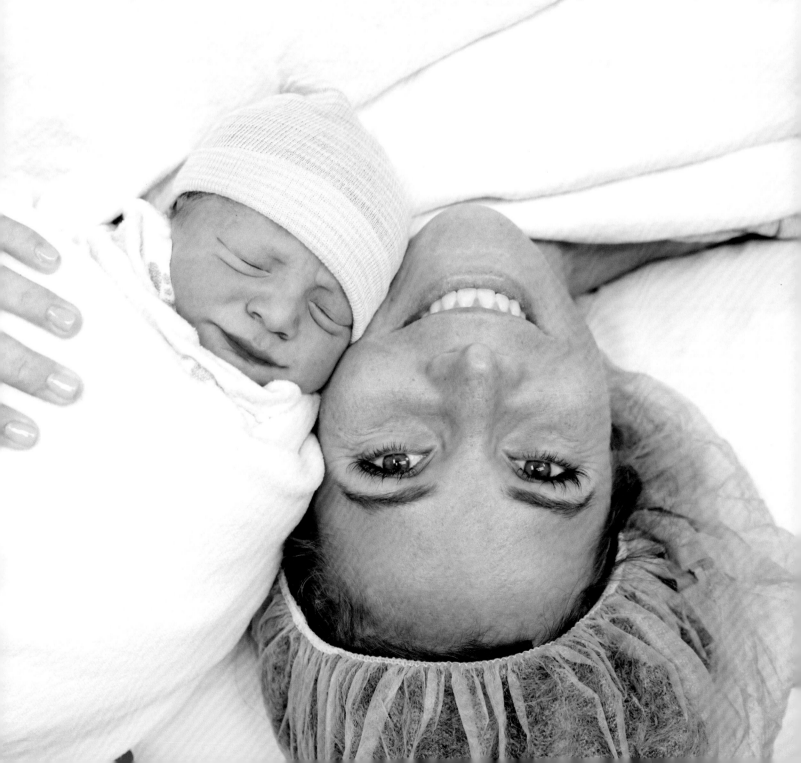

Reasons for a Cesarean Birth

In a cesarean birth, your baby is born through a surgical incision in your abdominal wall. Cesarean births are performed only when a vaginal birth is not possible or when there is concern for your well-being or the safety and health of your baby.

Reasons may include:

- Position of the baby.
- Prolonged labor.
- Placenta and cord problems.
- Fetal distress.
- Medical complications.
- Multiple *gestation* (twins, triplets, etc).

Position of the Baby

Face or Brow Presentation

A face or brow presentation is where the actual face or forehead (rather than the back portion of the head) presents first. There are some people who can give birth to a baby in these positions because of their pelvic outlet size or shape, but for some, this situation creates a problem.

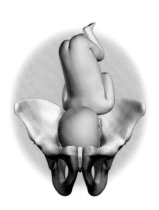

Transverse Lie

A horizontal position of the baby in the uterus is called a transverse lie. Almost all patients with babies in a transverse lie must have a cesarean birth.

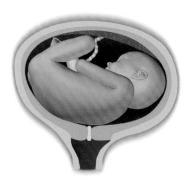

Breech Presentation

When the buttocks or feet, instead of the head, appear first, it is considered a breech presentation. The typical breech positions are illustrated below. Today, most people with a breech presentation in labor or breech position with ruptured membranes have a cesarean birth.

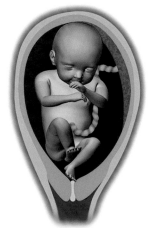
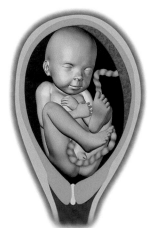
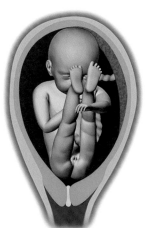

| Footling | Complete | Frank |

 Find supporting tools and videos in YoMingo.

Prolonged Labor

Prolonged labor occurs when your labor has stopped progressing during the first or second stage. What this means is that your cervix does not continue to dilate or efface, or your baby does not move into the birth canal. This stalled progression can be due to a variety of reasons such as ineffective contraction strength, the position of your baby's head, or the difference in the size of your pelvis and the size of your baby's head. Patience, augmentation of contraction strength, and purposeful repositioning are some solutions to help determine whether a cesarean birth may be appropriate.

Placenta and Umbilical Cord Complications

Placenta Previa

The placenta usually is attached to the upper uterine wall away from the cervix. In a placenta previa, the placenta is attached low on the uterine wall either partially or completely covering the cervical opening. Placenta previa usually shows up as painless bleeding. A sonogram can detect this issue early. The bleeding can be light or heavy and may initially appear in mid-pregnancy. Early delivery by cesarean birth may be necessary because of heavy bleeding that can cause fetal distress.

> Your healthcare provider will decide the safest route of birth for you and your baby.

Abruptio Placentae

If the placenta detaches from the wall of your uterus before your baby is born, it is called an abruption. This is a serious problem because the oxygen source to your baby can be compromised and you will be bleeding from the separated area. Constant pain and a hard, rigid abdomen can be a sign of abruption. An emergency cesarean is usually performed.

Prolapsed Umbilical Cord

Another true emergency is a prolapsed umbilical cord — the cord slides out of the cervix in front of your baby. This is a major problem and an emergency cesarean must be performed. When your uterus contracts and pushes your baby down, pressure on the umbilical cord can diminish the blood flow to your baby and may cause severe fetal distress. This does not happen often. It is most likely to occur if you are preterm, your baby is breech presentation, or your baby's head is not well-engaged into your pelvis when your water breaks.

Abruptio Placentae: detaches from the wall prematurely.

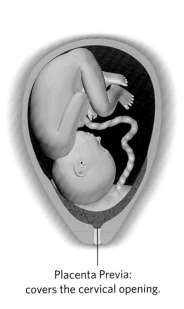

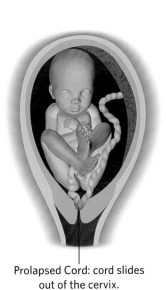

Placenta Previa: covers the cervical opening.

Prolapsed Cord: cord slides out of the cervix.

Fetal Distress

The umbilical cord can be wrapped around the baby's neck, looped around the body or caught between the baby's head and the bony pelvis. With a contraction, the cord may be pinched or stretched tightly so less oxygen is delivered to the baby. A fetal monitoring device can detect the problem. This can sometimes be relieved by simply changing your position. You are usually given oxygen and positioned on your left side. If the distress persists and is not relieved with any of the above techniques, then the healthcare provider will consider an assisted birth if the head is low enough in the pelvis. If it is not, a cesarean will be performed.

Complications

Any serious medical conditions you have that may complicate your health or jeopardize your baby's well-being by laboring are considered complications. These complications may require a cesarean birth.

Some conditions include:

- Very *premature infant*.
- A heart condition.
- Poorly controlled diabetes.
- Preeclampsia.
- High blood pressure.

- Active case of *genital herpes*.
- Multiple gestation (twins, triplets, etc).
- Rupture of membranes with signs of infection.
- Previous cesarean birth with a classical, or vertical, incision into the uterus.

Vaginal Birth After Cesarean (VBAC)

In the past, most thought that once someone had a cesarean birth, any future babies should also be delivered by cesarean. *Vaginal Birth After Cesarean (VBAC)* has evolved as an option, but it is not for everyone. VBAC can be accomplished in many instances and usually requires a shorter hospital stay. It can lead to a speedier recovery and an earlier return to normal activities. Cesarean births involve major surgery and some type of anesthesia. Infection, bleeding, and wound complications occur more frequently with cesarean births.

The first factor that is considered in the option for VBAC, sometimes called TOLAC or Trial of Labor After Cesarean birth, is the type of uterine incision that was used with your previous cesarean birth. The skin incision that you have on your abdomen is not necessarily in the same direction as your uterus, or womb, incision.

Your previous surgical records are used to evaluate this factor. Certain other factors may rule out an attempted VBAC, such as a breech position, above-average-sized baby and the location of the placenta. Many people who have had a previous cesarean birth may attempt VBAC since the benefits often outweigh the risks. Special medical precautions will be taken to protect both you and your baby. You will need an IV in your arm, and special monitoring will be performed on your baby to alert your healthcare provider of any signs of fetal distress.

VBAC may be an option for many people, but no labor and birth are risk-free. You should know the risks of VBAC and weigh these against the benefits before you decide. Many healthcare providers now offer TOLAC/VBAC as an option. If you are a candidate, both you and your healthcare provider should agree that it is a safe option. Consult with your healthcare provider about your individual circumstances.

Types of Uterine Incisions

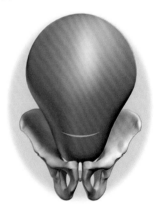

Low Transverse Incision

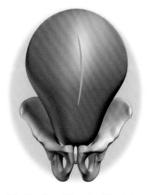

Vertical or Classical Incision

Cesarean Birth Procedure

Preparation for Cesarean

If a cesarean is necessary, your healthcare provider or the support staff will discuss the procedure and its indications along with options for anesthesia. The actual birth of the baby usually takes from 2 minutes, in an emergency, to 10 minutes in a non-emergency situation. Delivery of the placenta and closure of all the layers of the abdomen takes approximately 45 to 60 minutes.

- Lab work is drawn and IV is started.
- Hair is shaved around the incision site.
- Antacid and antibiotics are given.
- You are transferred to the operating room.
- Your support person waits in the preparation room until right before the surgery begins.
- Monitors are attached to you, and the anesthesia is administered.
- A urinary catheter is placed in your bladder.
- Sequential Compression Devices (SCD's) are placed on the lower legs to reduce risk of blood clots.
- The skin on your abdomen is washed and scrubbed with an antiseptic.
- Sterile drapes are placed.
- Your support person joins you.
- The surgery begins.

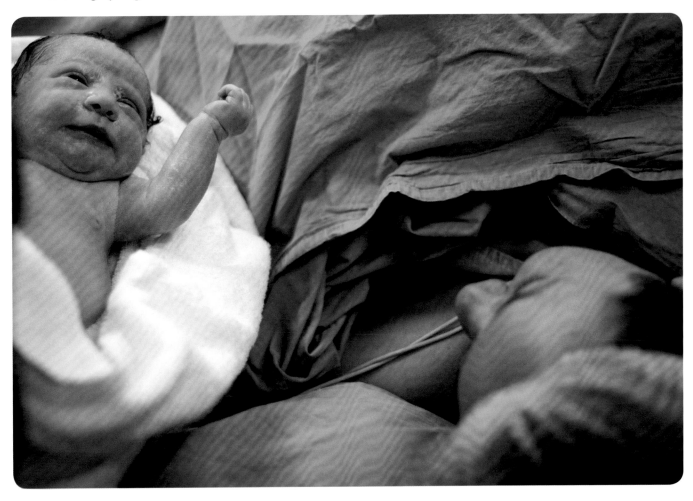

What Will I Feel During a Cesarean Birth?

Having surgery can be a scary idea, especially if you've never had surgery before. You may wonder if you will have any pain. Do not worry. Your healthcare team will make certain that you are comfortable and have enough anesthesia before beginning the surgery. What you will feel is pulling, tugging and pressure sensations. This is all normal and to be expected. There are also many sights, sounds and smells that you have probably never encountered before. If any of these cause you anxiety, your anesthesiologist is right by your head and can provide encouragement and support, as well as medications, if you need them. Remember the relaxation techniques that you practiced for labor. These tools can be used during a cesarean birth as well.

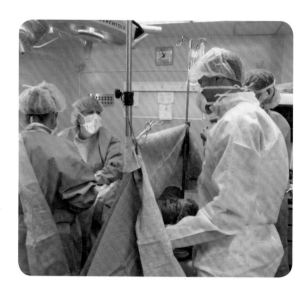

When Will I See My Baby?

During a "gentle" cesarean birth, a clear drape can be used in front of you so that you will be able to see your baby being born. If your newborn baby is doing well, they can be placed directly on your bare chest. Warm blankets will be placed over both of you to keep you warm. If your new baby needs some extra support following birth, they will be cared for in a warmer in the operating room. Your support person is welcome to go to the warmer and see the baby during this time. Once the surgery is completed, a healthy baby will go to the recovery room with you.

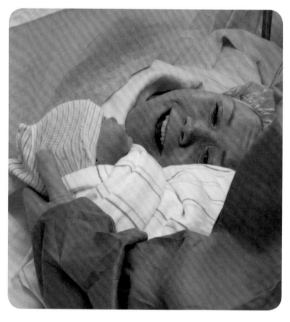

Immediate Post-Operative Recovery

Back in your recovery room, several monitors will assess how you are doing following surgery. Certain key actions and assessments will take place by your healthcare providers during this time.

- Pain management.
- Assessment of the amount of vaginal bleeding.
- Assessment of the incision site.

Pain Management

If you received a spinal or used an epidural for anesthesia during the surgery, you should be comfortable for several hours as it slowly wears off. If you received general anesthesia, however, post-operative pain management will be a priority in the recovery room. Tablets, injections or an IV attachment called a *patient-controlled analgesia*, or PCA, pump are all options to deliver pain relief. Through the PCA pump, pain medication can be administered continuously with the option for you to press a button that will deliver an extra amount of pain medication. Some healthcare providers choose to place a device in the incision site that delivers localized pain medication. Please be aware that there will be a level of pain that medication will not relieve during your recovery. Using your relaxation techniques that you learned for labor can be effective in relieving pain.

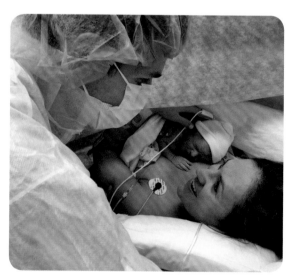

Assessment of Vaginal Bleeding

You may also need to use your relaxation techniques during recovery while your caregiver performs fundal massage. Just like with a vaginal birth, your uterus will be assessed for firmness and massaged, if necessary, to minimize vaginal bleeding. This action can be uncomfortable. Your caregiver will let you know before doing this assessment so you can prepare yourself.

Assessment of the Incision Site

Assessing your incision site will also be a priority. Unless your healthcare provider has opted to place a clear dressing on your incision, your recovery room caregiver will be assessing your bandage and not the actual incision. There are several different options for covering your incision, including transparent dressings and non-stick dressing pads used with flexible, highly breathable surgical tape. An advanced dressing that uses a vacuum to create negative pressure is often used for those with a high BMI, or body mass index. This dressing wicks away moisture to create a dry environment for the incision to heal.

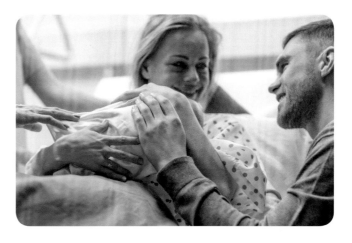

What Is Under That Bandage?

Please take note, your incision is not the size of your bandage. Once the dressing is removed you will see how your incision is being held together. Internal sutures, external staples, surgical glue, or wound closure strips are the typical forms of incision closure. Many healthcare providers simply choose the method they prefer. If you have a preference, please communicate that to your caregiver.

When Can I Eat?

During any surgical procedure the digestive system slows down significantly, leading to gas buildup and decreased bowel function. It is wise to wait until your intestines begin moving again before introducing any solid foods. When you are ready, getting up and moving will help this process. You will likely be given ice chips at first, followed by sips of water. Expect your diet to be advanced slowly while waiting for your intestines to "wake up."

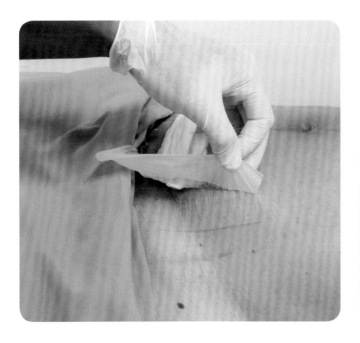

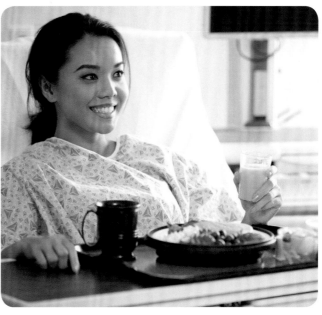

- **Pain with Coughing and Deep Breathing**
Because it is painful to take deep breaths and to cough following abdominal surgery, the tendency is to avoid it. Unfortunately, by not expanding your lungs and expelling any collected mucus, you are placing yourself in danger of further complications. To make this less painful, try taking a pillow and placing it over your incision. Gently but firmly put pressure against the pillow as if you are hugging it. This action is called "splinting" and it helps to provide support to your incision while you take deep breaths or cough. Please practice deep breathing and coughing following surgery. It is very important.

- **Incision Pain**
Practice "splinting" with a pillow before you move. This will help you provide more support to the incision site and make you feel more comfortable when changing positions. Pain medication helps as well.

- **IV Removal**
The IV will be removed when you can tolerate food.

- **Pain with Moving**
The sooner you get up and move around, the faster you will heal and the better you will feel. Your nurse will first have you sitting up on the side of the bed, then sitting in a chair and, finally, strolling in the hallway.

- **Urinary Catheter**
The urinary catheter, used to drain your bladder, will be removed once you are able to get out of bed and move around.

- **Vaginal Discharge**
Expect to have some bloody vaginal discharge after a cesarean birth. It will be bright red the first few days. It will then change to a deeper red color followed by a brown hue, and finishing with a somewhat yellow discharge. If you start to have active or bright red bleeding (more than a heavy period), passage of clots, or foul smell call your healthcare provider immediately.

Since a cesarean birth is major surgery, the recovery period will take longer than from a vaginal birth. It will also take a little longer for you to get back into your normal routine than from a vaginal birth. The usual hospital stay for cesarean birth is 48 to 72 hours. Discharge instructions for going home will be reviewed with you by your nurse or healthcare provider. Once you get home from the hospital, do not hesitate to call your healthcare provider with any questions.

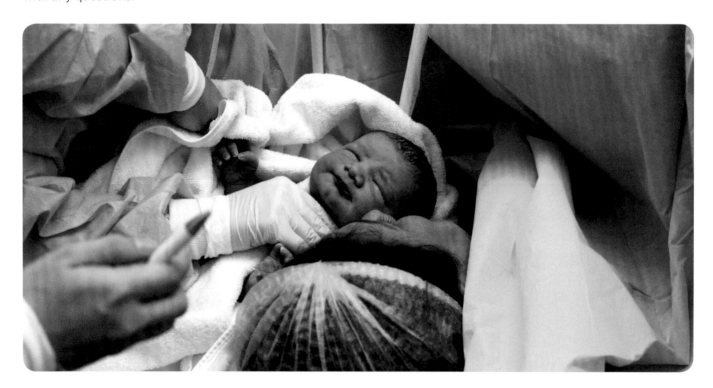

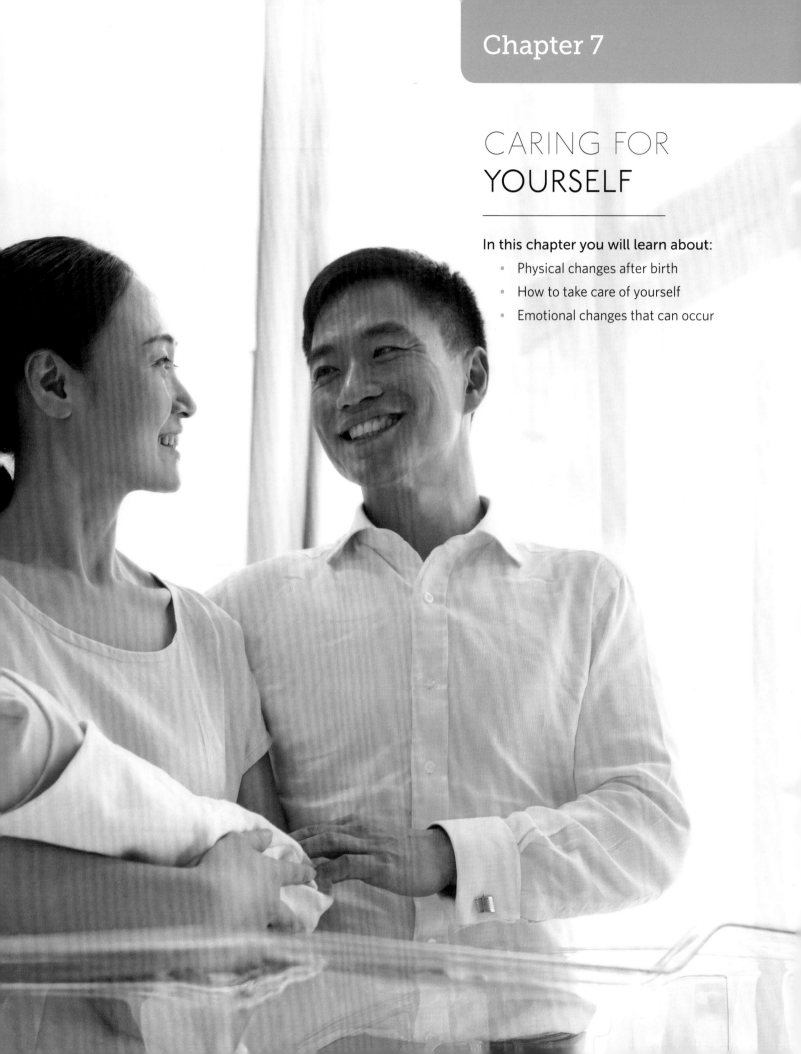

CARING FOR YOURSELF

In this chapter you will learn about:

- Physical changes after birth
- How to take care of yourself
- Emotional changes that can occur

Adjustment to Parenting

Being aware of your own physical and emotional well-being as you take your new infant home is very important during this special time. Do not be alarmed if the adjustment to parenting takes longer than you think. It is not only about recovering from the birth and figuring out how to take care of yourself, but also your new baby. There are things you need to adapt to that go well beyond that initial postpartum period.

Before you can feel like yourself again, your body needs to get back to normal, you need to regain a sense of control over your day-to-day routines, and you need to understand that your lifestyle is now completely different than it was before your baby arrived. You will start to rebuild your activities in a way that feels good and works for you and your family. This usually does not happen until your baby is in a routine and you are getting sleep and feeling more rested.

Tips to make your own care a top priority:

Get the rest and sleep you need when you need it.	This means you should accept help from family and friends. Allow others to take on some of the responsibilities associated with taking care of household chores. Accepting help is a good thing.
Get a break when you need it.	Every new parent deserves regular down time. Having a "break" is essential for managing fatigue and also for maintaining emotional health. Do not feel guilty for wanting or needing a break.
Get adequate exercise and nutrition.	You must continue to eat and maintain a well-balanced diet. Less sugar and processed foods, more grains, fresh fruits and vegetables are a part of healthy eating. Also getting your body moving is very important for emotional and physical well-being. Walking is very effective in the early weeks.

Physical Changes After Birth

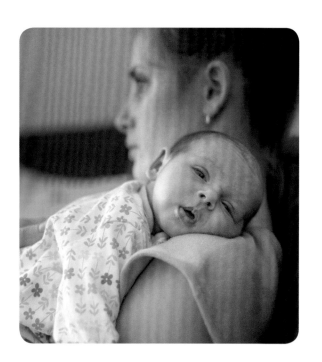

The first 6 weeks following the birth of your baby is called the postpartum period. These weeks are important as your body returns to a new normal after labor and birth. At the same time, you are welcoming a new life into your world. Knowing what to expect and relying on the continuing support of your healthcare team will help you relax in the postpartum experience with as much confidence and comfort as possible.

Your body gradually moves toward its pre-pregnancy state during these 4 to 6 weeks. The amount of time needed for this process varies, depending on the type of birth you had and other medical conditions.

The Uterus

The normal changes of the pregnant uterus to hold a developing baby are not reversed overnight. During pregnancy the uterus increases to about 11 times its non-pregnant weight. Right after birth it weighs more than 2 pounds and measures about the size of a grapefruit. It can be felt just below the bellybutton. In about 6 weeks the uterus will return to its normal weight of only 2 ounces.

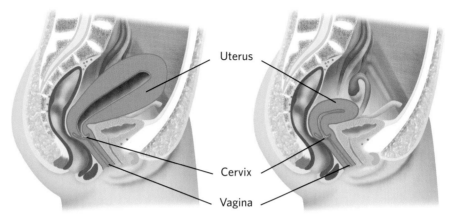

Uterus

Cervix

Vagina

Enlarged uterus after giving birth   Normal uterus size and position

Lochia (Vaginal Discharge)

You will have vaginal discharge while the area where the placenta was attached heals and the lining of the uterus is shed. This discharge, called *lochia*, is usually described as having a "fleshy, musty or earthy" smell. The smell should not be bad. You may notice your lochia is heavier when you stand up. This heavier flow is from the blood that collects in your vagina while you are sitting or lying down. Too much activity can also cause a heavier blood flow. This is your sign to slow down or rest. You may have less lochia if you had a cesarean birth. Wear pads until your lochia stops, not tampons. Tampons increase the chance for infection in your uterus.

First 2 to 3 days	About days 4 to 10	About days 10 to 21
• Bright to dark red.	• Pink or brown-tinged.	• Yellowish-white color.
• Heavy to medium flow.	• Medium to light flow.	• Very light flow.
• May have small clots.	• Very few or no clots.	• No clots, bright red color, or bad smell.

Be sure to tell your nurse or healthcare provider if you:

- Soak more than 1 pad an hour for 2 to 3 hours.
- Pass large clots or still have bright red bleeding after day 4.
- Notice your lochia has a bad smell.
- Have a fever over 100.4°F.
- Have severe pain in your lower abdomen.

Bowel Elimination

Hormones, medications, dehydration, perineal pain and decreased physical activity may make bowel function sluggish after birth. Your first bowel movement usually happens within 2 to 3 days. It may be a little uncomfortable, and you may be a little afraid.

When it is time	What can help
• Try to relax. • Put your feet up on a stool and rest your elbows on your knees. • From the front you can hold a clean sanitary pad over your perineum for support. • Avoid straining. It can make hemorrhoids worse.	• Don't resist the urge. • Drink 6 to 8 glasses of water a day. • Eat fiber-rich foods. • Keep moving — walk or do yoga stretches. • Take stool softeners.

Hemorrhoids

A hemorrhoid is a dilated blood vessel under the skin. They can be inside the rectum or outside on the anus. Hemorrhoids are not usually serious but can be painful.

Symptoms	What can help
• Pain or discomfort. • Itching. • Irritation. • Small amount of bleeding. • Swelling around the anus.	• Avoid straining during bowel movements. • Avoid sitting or standing for long periods of time. • Try cold compresses and/or warm baths. • Use pre-moistened wipes instead of toilet paper. • Use topical creams, suppositories and pain medication as directed by your healthcare provider.

Bladder

It is important for you to try to empty your bladder every 3 to 4 hours for the first few days after giving birth. Your bladder may become full and push on your uterus. This may keep your uterus from contracting and cause you to bleed more. Your body will be getting rid of extra fluid that caused hand and leg swelling late in pregnancy. You will notice that you have large amounts of urine the first few days at home.

If you had a cesarean birth:

You will have a catheter in your bladder during your first day after surgery. This will let you rest and allow your nurse to measure your urine output.

Be sure to tell your nurse or healthcare provider if you:

- Have a frequent or urgent need to urinate.
- Have severe pain or rectal bleeding.
- Feel you need a laxative.

Self-Care

It is best to get up and move around soon after birth, but exactly when you start depends on the type of birth experience you had. Moving around lowers the risk of blood clots in the veins of your pelvis, legs, ankles and feet. It also helps with better bladder and bowel function and lessens your pain or discomfort, even with a cesarean birth.

Perineal Care

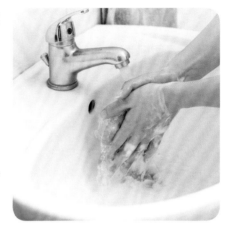

- Wash your hands often and carefully — both before and after changing sanitary pads.
- Wash your perineum with mild soap and water at least once daily.
- Rinse with lukewarm water 2 to 3 times daily and after urination and bowel movements.
- Wash and wipe from the front to back.
- Apply your pad from the front to the back.
- Change your pad every time after urinating or having a bowel movement.
- Check the amount and color of your lochia with each pad change.

Episiotomy Care

If you had an episiotomy it may take 4 weeks to heal. The sutures do not need to be removed because they will dissolve. Use a hand-held shower, a squeeze bottle or sitz bath to cleanse the episiotomy. Sometimes using antiseptic spray or analgesic cream can provide relief. Use moist antiseptic towelettes or toilet paper in a patting motion to dry the perineum. Please call if pain increases or becomes intense.

Cesarean Birth Incision

You may have staples closing your incision with a dressing over it. The dressing and the staples are removed before leaving the hospital or during a follow-up visit with your healthcare provider. Wound closure strips are put over your incision to help keep it closed. They will be very loose after several weeks. That's when you may gently remove them. It is important to check your incision daily.

> ⚠️ **Be sure to tell your healthcare provider if your incision becomes:**
> - Red
> - Separated
> - Swollen
> - Warm to touch
> - Tender or painful
> - Draining

Baths and Showers

Vaginal birth:

Showers are usually allowed as soon as your epidural catheter is removed and you walk well. Sitz or tub baths are generally safe after the second day. They are preferred by many because of discharge and the discomfort from an episiotomy.

Cesarean birth:

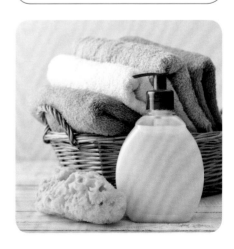

You may shower after the first day. Your healthcare provider will need to remove the dressing over your incision and your epidural catheter. Be sure you are able to stand and walk without getting dizzy. It is okay to get your incision wet. You may use soap on the upper part of your body and allow it to rinse down over your incision. Tub baths are not recommended for up to a few weeks after a cesarean birth. Check with your healthcare provider first to see when they recommend taking a tub bath.

Managing Postpartum Pain

Pain after birth depends on several factors: the length of your labor, the type of birth and your personal style of dealing with pain. In the first 1 to 2 days following childbirth, you will feel muscle aches and fatigue, particularly in your shoulders, neck and arms. This is a result of the physical exertion during labor. Joint stiffness in the hands is also common. This is a result of intravenous (IV) fluids given during labor and a natural redistribution of fluid.

As the uterus shrinks, its muscle fibers contract, causing *afterbirth cramps*. These mild contractions are most noticeable the first 3 to 4 days following birth. You may notice they are stronger when you are breastfeeding due to the hormones released during feeding. These contractions help to reduce blood loss and shrink the uterus to its pre-pregnancy state. There may be tenderness of the perineum. It may be worse if you had a tear or episiotomy.

Methods to Manage Pain

Comfort measures:

- Massage and relaxation.
- Deep breathing.
- Music.
- Ice packs for first 24 to 48 hours.
- Warm pad on abdomen for cramps.
- Warm sitz baths/herbal baths.

Medical pain relief options:

- Topical creams or sprays to specific areas.
- Over-the-counter medication like ibuprofen.
- Prescription medication.

Your nurse will review all your medications with you and explain their purpose, how often to take them and possible side effects. Most medications are compatible with breastfeeding. To be safe, check with your healthcare provider before taking over the counter or prescribed medications. Set your personal pain goal for pain management or identify the number on the rating scale at which you feel you need pain medication.

Pain Rating Scale

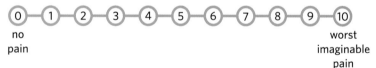

no
pain

worst
imaginable
pain

Please let your nurse know any time you have pain and need medication. Your nurse will ask you for your pain rating number before giving you pain medication. They will ask you again about an hour after you took it to check that it worked. Be sure to ask your nurse if you have any questions about the medications your healthcare provider has prescribed.

Be sure to tell your nurse or healthcare provider if your pain is:

- Constant.
- Unusual.
- Worse than it was before.
- Keeping you from doing things you were able to do before.
- Located in the right upper area of your abdomen or just below your breastbone.
- A headache with ANY vision changes OR confusion/mental changes OR dizziness OR new edema/swelling.

Managing your pain after a cesarean birth may be done through your epidural or IV tube until you can take pain pills. Some hospitals use PCA pumps (patient-controlled analgesia) that will allow you to control the medication you get by pushing a button. It is important that only you push the button. The pump is set according to the prescription from your doctor so you won't receive too much medicine.

Menstrual Cycle

Most people will have their first cycle within 7 to 9 weeks after giving birth. If you are breastfeeding you may not resume your menstrual period for 12 weeks or until you have completed breastfeeding. Egg production may return before the first menstrual period, which means you can become pregnant again.

Resuming Sex

Sexuality and recapturing closeness as a couple takes time. You and your partner may feel overwhelmed. You two should discuss resuming sex so that there will be few frustrations and misunderstandings. You may not be as interested in having sex as you were before pregnancy because of fatigue and the time demand by the baby. You may also have concerns about discomfort if you had a tear, episiotomy or cesarean incision. Tears and incisions can take a full 6 weeks to heal. You can expect vaginal dryness and reduced vaginal lubrication because of the hormones of pregnancy and/or breastfeeding. A water-based cream or jelly can solve this problem. If you experience difficulty with sexual intercourse, always discuss it with your partner. Set aside time for each other a few times each week without the baby to rebuild a satisfying sex life. Sharing feelings about sexuality is the most effective way to get back together both physically and emotionally.

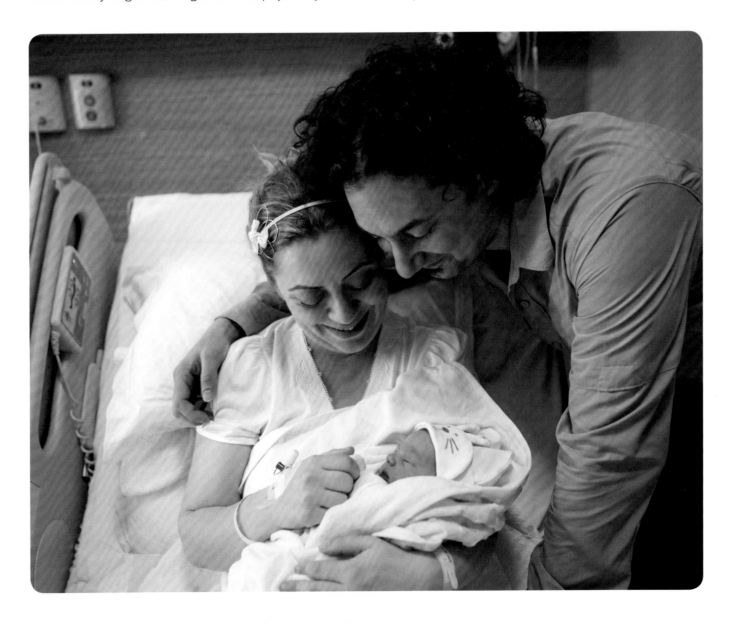

Emotional Changes

Along with the joy and relief of giving birth to your baby, you may experience sadness. You may find yourself crying, irritable, impatient, feeling a lack of confidence or inability to manage caring for yourself or your baby. Emotional changes can range from postpartum blues to clinical depression to psychotic depression. The difference lies in the nature and intensity of these feelings as well as how long they last. Studies have shown that new parents are more likely to develop these problems following the birth of their baby than at any other time in their lives.

Postpartum Blues

You may doubt yourself and your ability to be a good parent and take care of your new baby. You may:

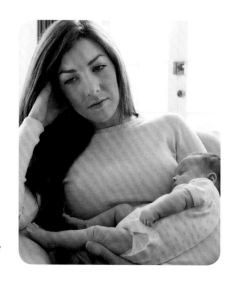

- Wonder what is wrong.

- Be tearful or easily irritated.

- Be anxious or ultra-sensitive.

- Be exhausted.

- Have trouble concentrating or sleeping.

- Feel overwhelmed by your responsibilities.

Such feelings occur in 9 out of 10 people who have given birth, whether this is their first or they have other children. The "blues" usually begin around the third or fourth day after birth and can last from a few hours to a week. Usually these feelings are short-lived and fade without any treatment.

Coping with Postpartum Blues

Keep your expectations realistic. Remember, you just gave birth to your baby. It takes time to learn about your baby and for your baby to learn about you.

- Rest as much as possible.

- Limit visitors.

- Allow others to do things for you.

- Let your partner know how you are feeling.

- If you are single, find and develop a good support system.

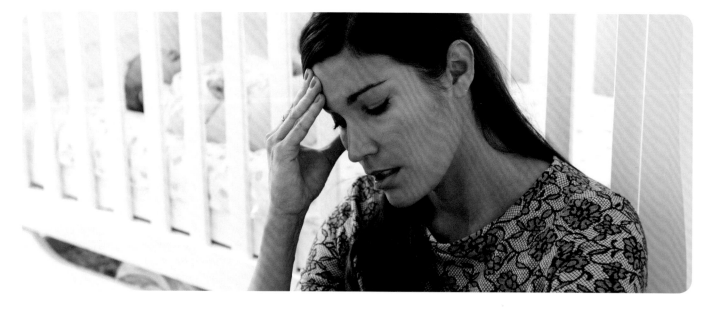

Postpartum Depression and Anxiety

When the "blues" last more than two weeks and get worse, you may have *postpartum depression or anxiety*. Many of the "blues" signs are present, but they are more severe or intense. This is not uncommon and happens to 1 to 2 of every 10 postpartum women. Postpartum depressive symptoms can appear any time during the first few months to one year after you give birth.

These feelings and experiences may lead you to become possessive of your baby or to disengage from and avoid your baby. This poses a risk to the physical and emotional safety of your baby. If untreated, these symptoms can last up to one year. There are several treatment options. Parents who get treatment usually respond extremely well.

Do not be afraid to be open and honest about how you are feeling. Your healthcare provider can help you connect with therapy, support groups, and other resources that can help you get better. You are not alone, and there is help for you.

Contact your healthcare provider if you have any of these signs or symptoms:

- Loss of identity.
- Complete loss of control.
- Feeling withdrawn, isolated and lonely.
- Change in appetite (either undereating or overeating).
- Exhausted, but unable to sleep.
- The need to keep moving or pacing.
- Mood swings.
- Constant crying.

- Constant anxiety or doubt.
- Difficulty sleeping or sleeping too much.
- Lack of interest in yourself, your baby or others.
- Overly concerned about cleanliness/germs and the health and safety of your baby.
- Feelings of hopelessness, a sense of failure or guilt.
- Feeling the need to "jump out of your skin".
- Nightmares.
- Difficulty focusing or concentrating.

Postpartum Psychosis

Below are some signs of postpartum psychosis. In very rare cases, a new parent can experience symptoms of psychosis. These symptoms usually start within 3 to 14 days after birth. A parent may not have all of them. Symptoms can vary or change quickly.

If a new parent has any of these symptoms they should be taken to the nearest emergency department and not be left alone with their baby.

- Can't remember how to do things they have done in the past or are extremely confused.
- Has a lot of energy, can't sleep, their mind keeps going.
- Has strange feelings, like something is crawling on them.
- Hears or sees things no one else does.

- Feels like someone else is controlling them.
- Agitation.
- Rapid or nonsense speech.
- They don't like how they feel and may be afraid.
- Has thoughts of harming themselves or their baby.

Find supporting tools and videos in YoMingo.

Postpartum Warning Signs:

It is normal to have discomforts like soreness and fatigue after you give birth. You may have other symptoms that could mean you need to see your healthcare provider or go to the nearest emergency room.

Contact your healthcare provider if you have any of these signs or symptoms:

- Bleeding that soaks a pad every hour for 2 to 3 hours.
- Bad smell coming from your vagina.
- Fever of 100.4°F or higher.
- Incision or abdominal pain that will not go away.
- Swelling, redness, discharge, or bleeding from your cesarean incision or episiotomy site.
- Your incision begins to separate.
- Problems urinating including inability to urinate, burning while urinating or extremely dark urine.
- No bowel movement within 4 days of giving birth.
- Any type of visual disturbance (double vision, blurring, etc).
- Severe headache.
- Excessive swelling of hands, feet or face.
- Flu-like symptoms.
- Pain or redness in one or both of your breasts.
- Pain, warmth, tenderness or swelling in your legs, especially the calf area.
- Frequent nausea and vomiting.
- Signs of depression or anxiety.

Call 911 if you have:

- Bleeding that is not controlled or stopping.
- Chest pain.
- Trouble breathing.
- Sudden onset of arm or leg weakness.
- Sudden facial drooping (may be on one side).
- Slurred speech, trouble speaking or are unable to speak.
- Chills, clammy skin, dizziness, fainting, racing heartbeat.
- Dramatic emotional changes like insomnia, severe agitation, confusion.

Do not ignore any of the symptoms below. You may think they are nothing, but they could mean something more.

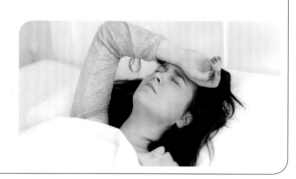

- Headache.
- Blurry or double vision, flashing spots or lights.
- Extra swelling in your hands, feet or face.
- Pain in your upper abdomen.

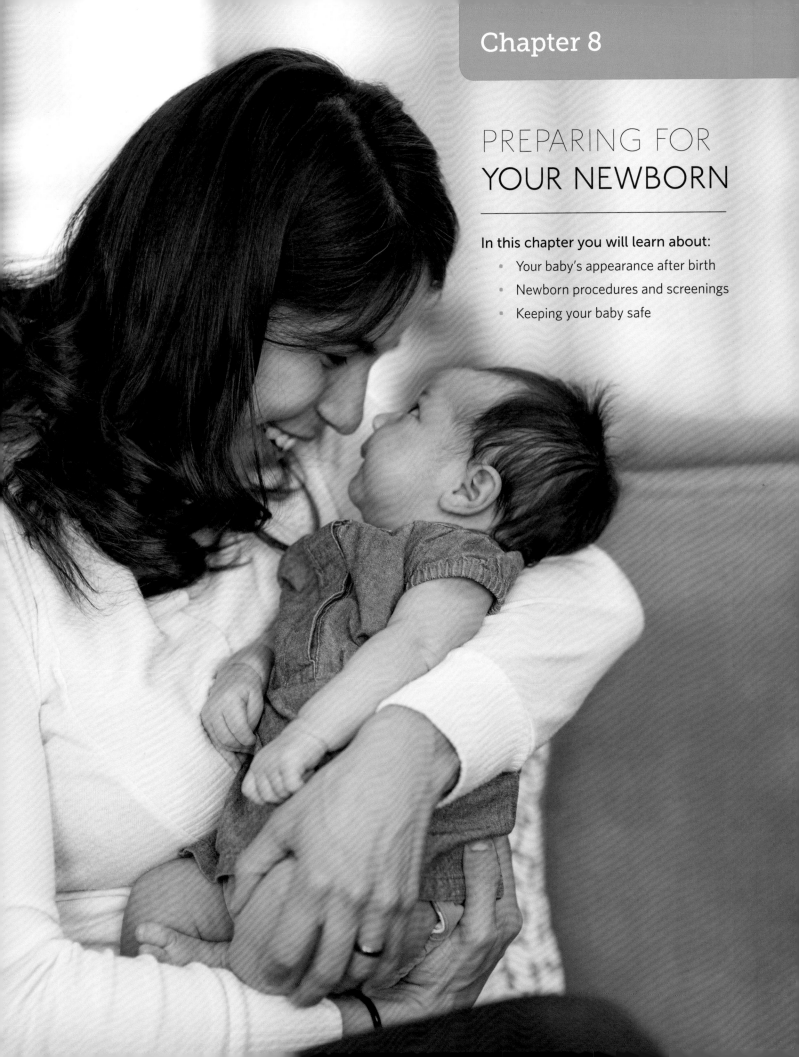

Chapter 8

PREPARING FOR YOUR NEWBORN

In this chapter you will learn about:

- Your baby's appearance after birth
- Newborn procedures and screenings
- Keeping your baby safe

Skin-to-Skin Contact

At birth, your baby may be placed directly on your chest. While you are holding your baby skin-to-skin, a member of the healthcare team will dry your baby. They will check your baby over and cover both of you with a warm blanket. Now the bonding can begin. This connection of your bare-skinned baby lying directly on your skin is called skin-to-skin contact and can give you and your baby time to get to know each other. This initial snuggling also has very important health benefits.

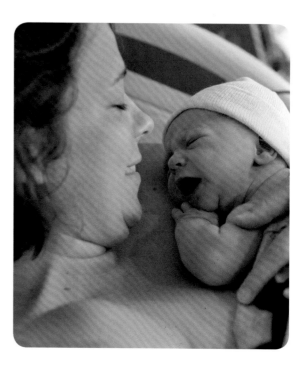

According to the American Academy of Pediatrics (AAP), the best start for breastfeeding is when a baby is kept skin-to-skin immediately after birth and until the first feeding has finished, or as long as the parent wishes. The baby's sense of smell allows them to find the breast to begin the initial latch-on. Research has shown that babies placed skin-to-skin after their birth breastfeed better and stay awake during the feeding. In addition, babies who had skin-to-skin contact are more likely to exclusively breastfeed. Regardless of how you plan to feed your baby, skin-to-skin is best practice for all babies.

Benefits of skin-to-skin contact

- Soothes and calms you and your baby.
- Helps your baby regulate their temperature, heart rate, breathing and blood sugar.
- Enhances bonding.
- Supports breastfeeding.
- Helps your uterus contract.

Proper position for safe skin-to-skin contact

- You should be semi-reclined or upright and alert, or have an alert adult at the bedside helping.
- Your baby is high up on your chest in a "kissable" position and laying in the middle of your chest.
- Your baby's head is turned to one side with mouth and nose visible and chin in a neutral position (not slouched).
- Your baby's arms and legs are flexed and held tight to the sides of their body.

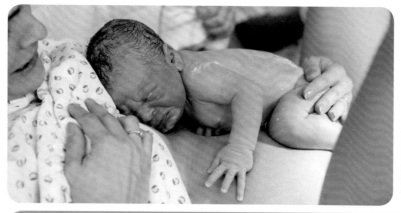

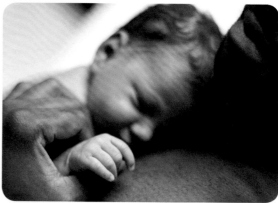

Remember: Babies should always maintain good skin color and respond to stimulation. Babies are usually calm and relaxed while skin-to-skin. Babies receive these benefits from being skin-to-skin with anyone, so allow other family members to bond with the baby this way, too.

 Find supporting tools and videos in YoMingo.

Apgar Score

The *Apgar test* is a quick and simple test your healthcare providers use to evaluate your baby's well-being at 1 minute and again at 5 minutes after birth. Your baby scores points in the 5 areas outlined in the chart. Most healthy babies average a score of 7 to 9.

Five Areas Evaluated	Points Given for Apgar Score		
	0	1	2
Heart Rate	Absent	Under 100	Greater than 100
Color	Blue to Pale	Body pinking — feet and hands blue	Pink
Breathing	Absent	Not regular	Crying/good rate
Muscle Tone	Absent/flaccid	Some movement	Active movement
Reflexes	No response to stimulation	Grimace	Sneeze or cough — responds to stimulation

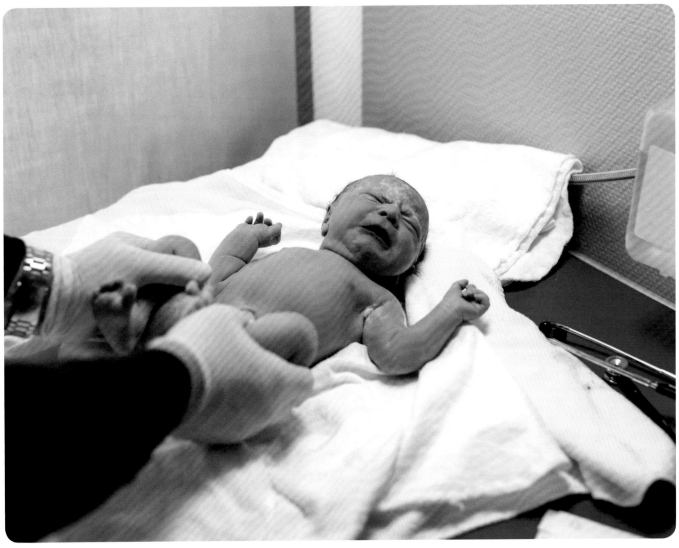

Your Baby's Appearance

As your baby is placed on your chest and dried off you will notice many characteristics about your baby. They are wet, tiny little human beings when they come into the world. What is amazing is how your baby's appearance changes in the hours and days after birth.

Color

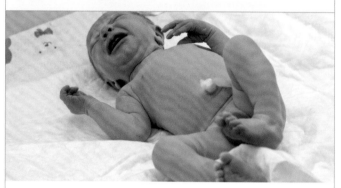

The first thing you might notice is your baby's color. Your baby's skin color will look bluish-gray at birth. This is normal. As your baby breathes and oxygen starts to circulate throughout their system you will notice their skin, lips, mucous membranes and nail beds becoming pinker. Your baby's hands and feet may appear to be bluish or purple in color at birth. This is called *acrocyanosis* and is also normal. Each baby is so different. Your baby's skin tone may continue to change in the weeks ahead.

Head Shape (Molding)

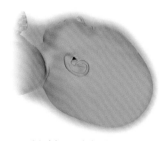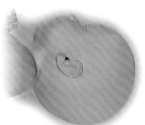

Molding of the head　　　Appearance days later

The plates of your baby's skull bones are not fused together. They are designed to allow a baby's head to change shape as they move through the narrow birth canal. They also accommodate your baby's rapidly growing brain during infancy. You may notice at birth that your baby's head looks out of shape. This is referred to as *molding*. You will find two areas known as soft spots on your baby's head. There is one at the top and one at the back where the skull bones have not yet grown together. These spots are called *fontanelles*.

Lanugo

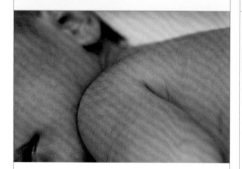

Some infants, especially those born before their due date, may be covered with fine hair. This is called *lanugo*. It grows on babies as they develop in the womb and provides additional skin protection. Lanugo disappears within a few weeks after birth.

Eyes

You might be surprised at how alert your baby is at birth. While they may turn their head toward the direction of different sounds, they can only see about 8 to 10 inches away. That is likely why they prefer looking mostly at your face. As their vision improves, they can see objects with contrasting

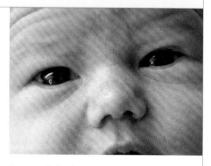

colors, like black-and-white patterns, the best. A baby's eyes are typically gray-blue or brown in color. You will not know what the true color will be for 9 to 12 months.

You may also see your baby's eyes cross sometimes. This is normal and will usually correct itself within 3 to 4 months. If your baby has red spots in the whites of their eyes, do not worry. These spots are simply broken blood vessels from the birth process and will disappear in the first week or two. They will have no lasting effects on your baby's sight.

Milia

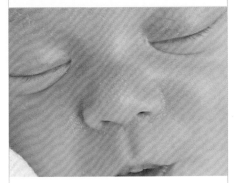

The nose of your baby may appear flat and may also be covered with *milia*. These are small, white, pimple-like bumps that are immature oil glands. You may also notice milia on the cheeks and forehead of your baby. Do not squeeze or pick at them. They will go away without treatment.

Vernix

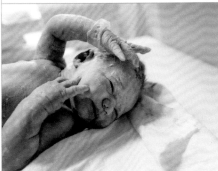

Your baby may be covered in a thick, white, cheesy coating called *vernix*. Although it might look strange, vernix is an amazing substance that protects your baby's skin. While floating in amniotic fluid for months, vernix keeps your baby's skin from becoming wrinkled. If vernix is present, this coating gets absorbed into the skin quickly after birth.

Mongolian Spots

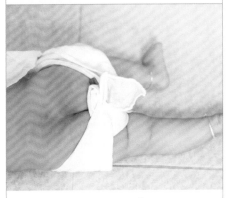

Mongolian spots are flat birthmarks that are very common among dark-skinned babies of Native American, African, Asian or Hispanic descent. They can be deep brown, slate gray or blue-black in color. These spots are sometimes mistaken for bruising but are not related to that in any way. Some marks can be small, and others can be up to 6 inches or more in diameter. They are usually found on the shoulders, lower back or buttocks area and will often fade after the first year of life.

Swollen Breasts and Genitals

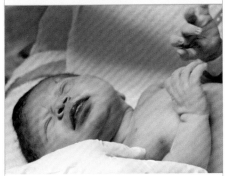

Babies' breasts and genitals may look a little swollen in both boys and girls. The breasts may also secrete a small amount of fluid. This is normal and caused by your hormones. After a few days the swelling will go away. Little girls may have a small amount of blood-tinged discharge. This, too, is normal. It is also due to hormones and may be noticeable in their diaper.

Dry Skin

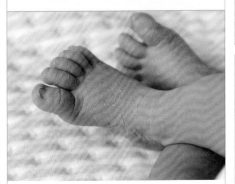

Babies born after their due date can be born with dry, wrinkly skin. The vernix, or protective coating on the skin, starts to slough off around 38 weeks of pregnancy, and after 40 weeks there may not be much left on the skin. Dry skin improves quickly in the days after birth as a baby's underlying skin is moist and healthy.

Stork Bites

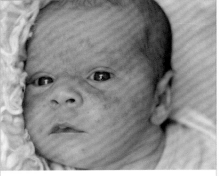

Stork bite is a playful name for birthmark. Babies are born with an assortment of common marks on their bodies. These are small red or pink patches that will usually disappear within the first year of life.

Procedures

The following procedures are commonly done in the first few days of your baby's life. Many parents are requesting in their birth plans that some procedures are omitted or delayed, so discuss them with your healthcare provider.

Eye Treatment

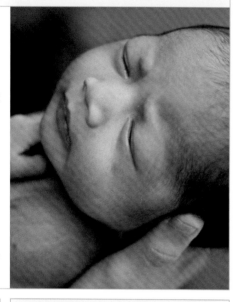

Health organizations recommend that all newborns receive eye treatment to protect them from infection. Antibiotic ointment, such as erythromycin, is applied in the infant's eyes immediately after birth to kill or weaken bacteria, especially the one causing gonorrhea. If left untreated, gonorrhea can cause eye damage and blindness. This ointment also offers protection against less serious types of pink eye caused by the sexually transmitted infection chlamydia or by other bacteria.

Some pregnant people make an informed decision to delay or forgo the antibiotic treatment. To consider this option you should have negative results of gonorrhea and chlamydia screenings during pregnancy, along with a monogamous relationship with an uninfected partner. It is important to discuss this decision with your healthcare provider early as some states in the U.S. have laws requiring the erythromycin treatment for all newborns. Become informed early so you can make the right decision for your family.

Identification

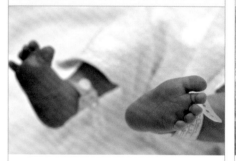

Most hospitals use a 4-band system with a number or barcode for identification. One bracelet will be placed on your wrist, two on your baby (the ankle and wrist) and one on another person you choose. Some hospitals also use tags that go on both you and your baby that include computerized chips, or radio frequency identification (RFID) tags. Many hospitals also use tamper-resistant alarms with embedded technology to help keep your baby safe.

Circumcision

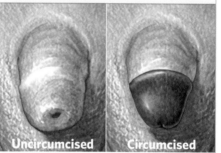

Uncircumcised   Circumcised

Circumcision is the removal of foreskin that surrounds the head of the penis. The American Academy of Pediatrics states the health benefits outweigh the risk of the procedure, however the benefits are not great enough to recommend neonatal circumcision. Discuss the benefits and risks with your healthcare provider and make an informed decision. The choice of circumcision is a personal one and may be based on religious, cultural or traditional factors.

Vitamin K

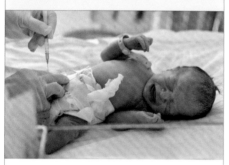

Vitamin K helps with blood clotting. Babies are born with only a small amount of vitamin K, so they are at risk for vitamin K deficiency bleeding (VKDB). Bleeding can develop spontaneously from an unknown cause, or there may be an underlying disorder causing bleeding. An injection of vitamin K is given in the baby's thigh immediately after birth. Some parents prefer to have the injection given while the baby is held skin-to-skin or breastfeeding to minimize any pain.

Newborn Screenings

Newborn screenings test infants shortly after birth for medical conditions that are treatable, but not seen, in the newborn period. Every state in the U.S. requires certain newborn screening tests on all babies.

Metabolic Screening

Metabolic screening is an essential preventive health measure. It tests for developmental, genetic and metabolic disorders in the newborn. These conditions may not be apparent immediately after birth. If identified early, many of these rare conditions can be treated before they cause serious health problems. Each state requires screening, but the specific test done may vary. Some disorders are more common in some states, making these screenings even more important.

How the test is performed:

A few drops of blood are taken from your baby's heel. This is usually done on the day of discharge or no later than 2 to 3 days after birth. The sample is then sent to the lab for testing. Make sure the hospital and your baby's healthcare provider have your contact information so you can be notified of the results.

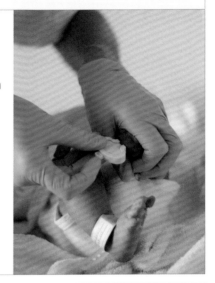

Hearing Screening

Of every 1,000 babies born, it is estimated that 1 to 3 will have serious hearing loss. Hearing screening for newborns before they leave the hospital or maternity center is becoming a common practice. It is recommended that all newborns be screened for hearing. If hearing loss is not caught early on, there will be a lack of stimulation of the brain's hearing center. This can delay speech and other development in your newborn.

How the test is performed:

This test is painless and is performed using a tiny earphone, microphone or both while you are still in the hospital. The test takes about 10 minutes and is done while your baby is sleeping.

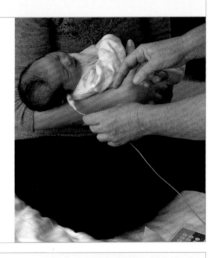

Pulse Oximetry Screening for Congenital Heart Disease

Pulse oximetry is a simple, painless test used to measure how much oxygen is in your baby's blood. It is done when your baby is more than 24 hours old. It is useful in screening for some congenital heart diseases in newborns.

How the test is performed:

Sensors are placed on the baby's hand and foot with a sticky strip and a small red light or probe. These sensors measure the baby's oxygen level and pulse rate. The test takes a few minutes to perform while the baby is still, quiet and warm.

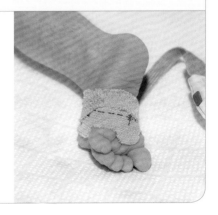

Jaundice ↻

Jaundice is common in newborn babies. It gives a yellow color to the baby's skin and eyes. Newborn babies have produced extra red blood cells for the birth process. One of the breakdown products of red blood cells is *bilirubin*. The liver in the newborn is fully developed, but not 100 percent efficient. Therefore, extra bilirubin in the blood is stored in the skin until the liver is able to break it down. This buildup of bilirubin in the blood and skin is called physiologic jaundice.

Most cases of jaundice will go away without any medical treatment. Your baby's healthcare provider will monitor the bilirubin level and treat it if it is too high. You may need to make extra visits to the healthcare provider's office or the lab in order to be certain that the bilirubin level is within an acceptable range. Left untreated, high levels of bilirubin can cause serious complications. It is important to take jaundice seriously and follow the instructions for appointments and recommended care.

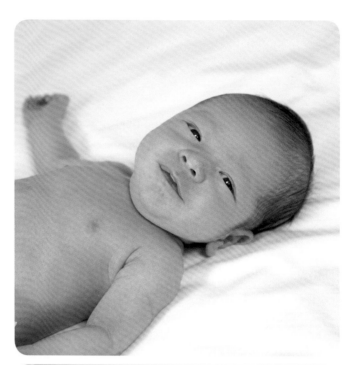

How the test is performed:

Transcutaneous bilirubin testing is a painless test done by placing a light meter on the baby's skin. If the bilirubin level is high, a blood test can be done. A small sample of blood from the baby's heel will be taken to measure the serum bilirubin levels. If these levels are high based on the baby's age in hours and other risk factors, treatment will be ordered.

Treatment

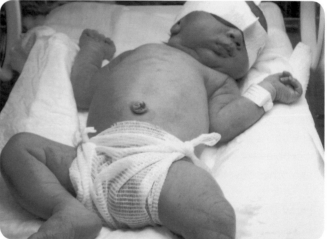

Phototherapy is treatment with a special light. The baby will be placed under the light wearing only a diaper and special eye protection. The lights will not hurt the baby. Another option for treatment is a fiberoptic blanket under the baby. The light and blanket are sometimes used together. The bilirubin levels will be checked by a blood test to ensure the treatment is working. Treatment can be done in the hospital or even at home.

Make sure your baby is getting enough to eat. Babies will get rid of the bilirubin through the stool. Breastfeed your baby 8 or more times a day for the first few days. This will help you make enough milk for the baby and will help keep the baby's bilirubin level down.

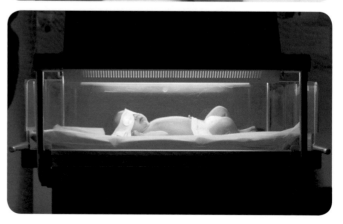

↻ Find supporting tools and videos in YoMingo.

Keeping Your Baby Safe

Rooming-In

Rooming-in (keeping parents and babies together in the same room) is beneficial to the health and development of infants. For you and your spouse or partner, the benefits of rooming-in include:

- You can respond and begin feedings promptly as you learn your baby's feeding cues.
- Your baby cries less and you can soothe them quickly.
- You make more breast milk, as breastfeeding occurs early and often.
- You get more rest.
- You gain confidence in caring for your baby while experienced staff is available.
- Your baby can be monitored easily.

Rooming-in is so valuable the AAP encourages parents to also do it at home. Rooming-in until your baby is at least 6 months old (ideally, 1 year) is part of the AAP's strategies for preventing SIDS.

Unless there is a medical issue with either you or your baby that requires you to be apart, rooming-in allows the hospital staff to care for you both at the same time.

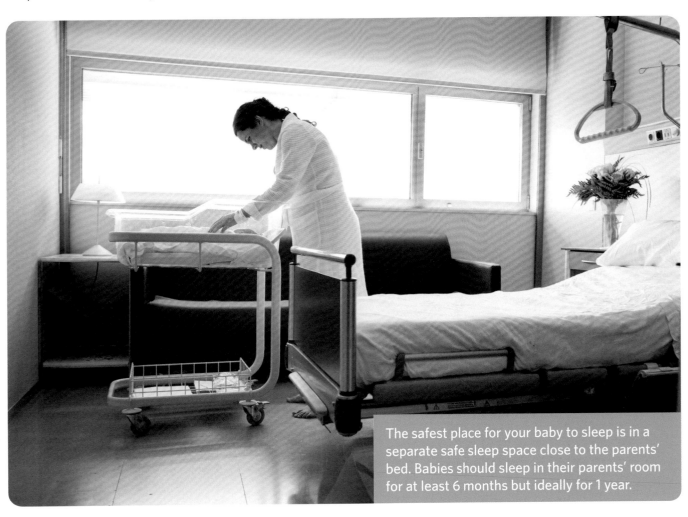

The safest place for your baby to sleep is in a separate safe sleep space close to the parents' bed. Babies should sleep in their parents' room for at least 6 months but ideally for 1 year.

Safe Sleep

The Centers for Disease Control and Prevention (CDC) estimates that nearly 3,500 infants die suddenly and unexpectedly each year in the United States. These deaths are called Sudden Unexpected Infant Deaths, or SUIDs. About half of all SUID deaths are due to Sudden Infant Death Syndrome, or SIDS, which are sudden deaths that cannot be explained. SIDS is the leading cause of SUID for infants under 1 year old, especially from birth to 4 months.

One of the best ways to reduce the risk of SIDS is to put healthy infants on their backs when putting them down to sleep at nighttime or naptime. Ever since the American Academy of Pediatrics (AAP) recommended that all babies be placed on their backs to sleep in 1992, deaths from SIDS have declined dramatically.

Sleep-related deaths from other causes, however, including suffocation, entrapment and asphyxia, have gone up. The safest place for a baby to sleep is on a separate sleep surface designed for babies that is close to the parents' bed. The AAP has given recommendations for a safe sleeping environment. Parents and caregivers, follow these important steps to help to protect your baby from SIDS and SUID.

| Make sure nothing covers the baby's head. | Dress your baby in sleep clothing, such as a one-piece sleeper, and do not use a blanket. | Always place your baby on their back to sleep, for naps and at night. | Keep pillows, sheepskins, crib bumpers and toys out of your baby's sleep area. |

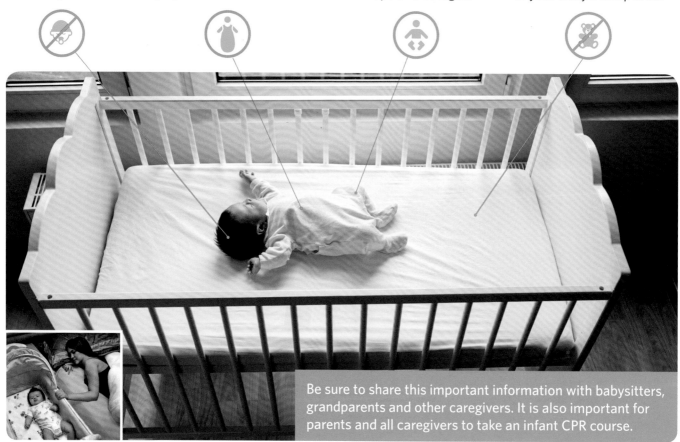

Be sure to share this important information with babysitters, grandparents and other caregivers. It is also important for parents and all caregivers to take an infant CPR course.

| Baby's sleep area is next to where parents sleep. Do not share a bed with your baby. | Do not smoke or let anyone smoke around your baby. | Use a firm sleep surface, such as a mattress in a safety approved crib, covered by a fitted sheet. |

Shaken Baby Syndrome

If you are a parent of a new baby, there may be times when you will become frustrated and maybe even angry when your baby cries. You may have tried everything to comfort them, but nothing seems to help. You are not getting any sleep and you may be very frustrated. No matter how you feel, do not shake your baby.

Shaken Baby Syndrome (SBS) or Abusive Head Trauma (AHT) is what happens when a baby is violently shaken. The movement of the baby's head back and forth can cause bleeding and increased pressure on the brain. A baby's neck muscles are not strong enough and the brain is too fragile to handle this "whiplash" motion. SBS is one of the leading forms of child abuse. Many babies die. Many others have irreversible brain damage. Those who survive may have visual disturbances or blindness, mental injury, paralysis, seizure disorders, learning and speech disabilities, or neck and back damage.

If you are feeling like you cannot deal with your baby's crying and you have met the baby's basic needs (clean diaper, fed, appropriate clothes, gently rocked, held, etc.) then STOP, think and reach out for help if you need it. There may be times when nothing you do will stop the crying. This is normal. DO NOT SHAKE YOUR BABY. If you think your baby has been shaken, take them to the emergency room immediately.

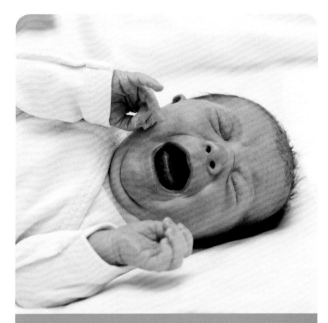

If you or a caregiver has violently shaken your baby because of frustration or anger, the most important step you can take is to SEEK MEDICAL ATTENTION IMMEDIATELY. Do not let fear, shame or embarrassment keep you from doing the right thing. Getting the necessary and proper treatment right away may save your child's life.

Signs and symptoms of Shaken Baby Syndrome include:

- Irregular, difficult or stopped breathing.
- Very fussy.
- Seizures or vomiting.
- Hard to feed.
- Hard to stay awake.
- No smiling or vocalization.
- Not able to focus or track movement with his eyes.

What to do if you get frustrated:

- NEVER THROW OR SHAKE YOUR BABY NO MATTER WHAT.
- Take a breath.
- Close your eyes and count to 10.
- Put your baby down in their crib and leave for a few minutes to calm down.
- Give yourself a "timeout."
- Ask a trusted friend, neighbor or family member to take over for a while.
- Do not pick the baby up until you feel calm.
- If you think they are sick, call your healthcare provider right away or take your baby to the hospital.

Car Seat Safety

Your baby needs a safe car seat to go home from the hospital. Every state requires that infants and children ride buckled up. The "best" car safety seat is one that fits your newborn and can be set up correctly in your car. Even the most expensive car seat may not protect your baby if it is not installed properly.

Using a car safety seat correctly can help prevent injuries to your infant. Never place an infant in a rear-facing seat in front of an active airbag. In most cars, the safest place is in the middle of the back seat.

To properly secure a child in a rear-facing seat:

- Place rolled blankets at each side of their head for positioning (if needed).
- Baby's head must be 1 inch below the top of car seat shell.
- Harness straps must be snug. You should not be able to pinch any slack in the harness at baby's shoulders.
- Do not attach toys, wraps, rides etc. to the car seat.
- Put a rolled blanket between baby and crotch strap (if needed).
- Tightly install child seat in the car's back seat, facing the rear. The infant seat should not move more than 1 inch side-to-side at the seatbelt pathway.
- Harness slots should be at or below baby's shoulders.
- Place harness retainer clip at armpit/nipple level.
- Avoid bulky clothing under the snug harness. Place a blanket over the child after they are securely strapped into in the car seat.
- Infant seat should recline at about a 45-degree angle.

Baby's Warning Signs

Even experienced parents may feel worried as they adjust to a new baby's habits, needs and personality. Remember that most of the common physical problems that occur during a given 24 hours with a baby may be normal situations or problems with simple answers.

Contact your healthcare provider if your baby has any of these signs or symptoms:

- **Blue lip color is a 911 call!**
- Blue or pale-colored skin.
- Yellow skin or eyes.
- Patches of white found in your baby's mouth.
- Eating poorly or refusing to eat.
- No stool for 48 hours and less than 6 wet diapers a day.
- Redness, drainage or foul odor from the umbilical cord.
- Does not urinate within 6 to 8 hours of circumcision.
- Temperature of 100.4°F or more.
- Difficulty breathing.
- Very fussy.
- Repeated vomiting or several refused feedings in a row.
- Listlessness or is hard to wake up.
- Crying excessively with no known cause or an unusual or high-pitched cry.
- An unusual or severe rash (other than prickly heat).
- Frequent or successive bowel movements with excess fluid, mucus or unusually foul odor.
- Signs of dehydration:
    - Dry or cracked lips.
    - Dry skin.
    - Dry or rough tongue.
    - Increased sleepiness or irritability.

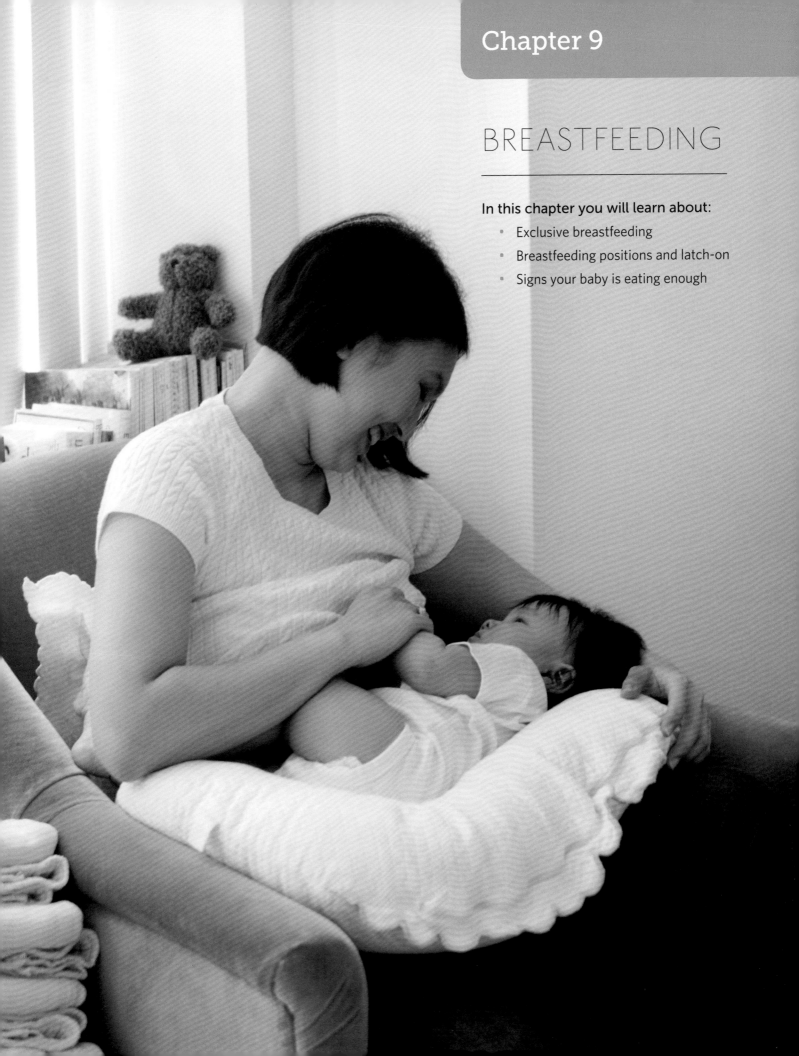

Chapter 9

BREASTFEEDING

In this chapter you will learn about:

- Exclusive breastfeeding
- Breastfeeding positions and latch-on
- Signs your baby is eating enough

Breastfeeding Benefits

By choosing to breastfeed you are providing the best source of nutrition for your baby. The benefits a baby receives from human milk will last a lifetime.

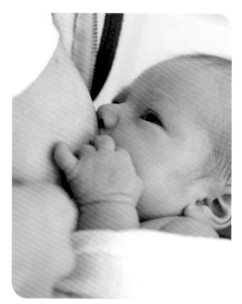

For your baby:

- Lower risk of Sudden Infant Death Syndrome (SIDS).
- Protects against respiratory and diarrheal disease.
- Reduces ear infections.
- Decreases obesity later in childhood.
- Less likely to have insulin-dependent diabetes.
- Decreases risk of childhood cancer.
- Protects against allergies.

For you:

- Lowers risk of osteoporosis later in life.
- Reduces risk of breast, uterine, endometrial and ovarian cancer.
- Decreases insulin use in a diabetic breastfeeding parent.
- Hormone release helps your uterus contract to prevent bleeding.

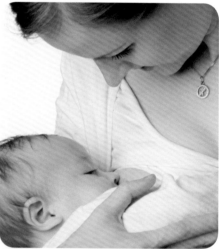

Note:

- Breast milk has all of the nutrients your baby needs.
- Breast milk contains antibodies to help your baby fight off viruses and bacteria.
- Breast milk protects your baby's gut from germs and diseases.
- Breastfeeding promotes bonding and contributes to your baby's emotional development.

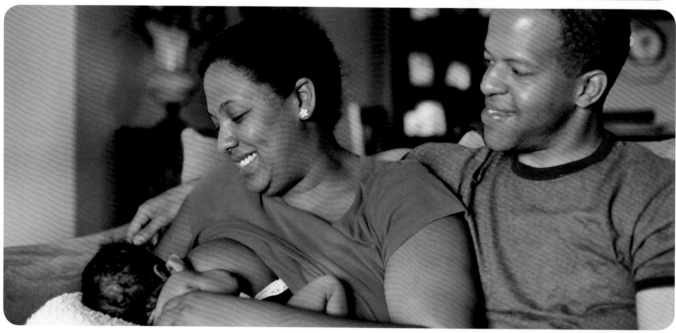

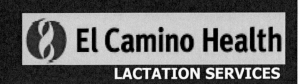
Supplemental Nursing System or "SNS"

- Supplemental feedings are hand expressed/pumped breast milk or formula that is given when a baby has difficulty latching on to the breast, mom cannot breastfeed, or the Doctor orders because of a medical condition.
- Hand express/pump both breasts after each time a supplement is given. Save milk for the next feeding.
- Breast milk is safe at room temperature for approximately 4-6 hours and in the refrigerator for 5-7 days.

Appropriate Amounts to Supplement Your Baby for Each Feeding (30 mls = 1 ounce)

Day 1	Day 2	Day 3	Week 1	Week 2	Week 3
5-7 mls	7-15ml	22-30 mls	30-45 mls	45-60 mls	~90 mls

GETTING ENOUGH MILK MEANS:
- Listening for swallows
- Counting the appropriate amount of wet/soiled diapers
- And baby gaining ½ to 1 ounce of weight after day 3-5.

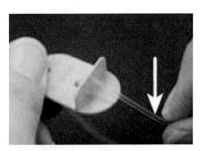

HOW TO USE SNS STARTER KIT *(from SNS manual):*
1. **Fill container with milk/formula**
2. **Press white membrane onto the upper side of the disc.**
3. **Place disc into Reservoir/Tubing assembly** so white membrane faces tubing. Click into place.
4. **Screw the Reservoir/Tubing assembly onto the container.**
5. **Turn the bottle upside down and gently squeeze reservoir** to allow a small amount into the reservoir.
6. **Close off tubing using Tubing Clamp** to avoid milk leaking. **Open clamp after latching.**
7. **Clip the bottle to your shirt no higher than the baby's head** or the milk may flow too quickly
   Watch carefully for milk spilling out of the baby's mouth, choking or "coughing" sounds from the baby.
8. **Tape tubing lengthwise onto your breast** about 1 inch from the tip of your nipple in the direction of the nose.
9. **It takes about 10-20 minutes** for the baby to take 1 ounce (30 mls).

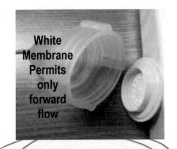

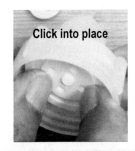

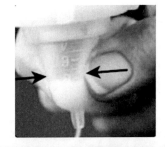

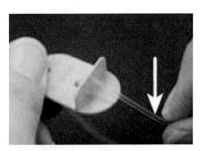

2485 HOSPITAL DRIVE
MOUNTAIN VIEW, CA 94040
650-988-8290

815 POLLARD ROAD
LOS GATOS, CA 95032
408-871-7479

WWW.ELCAMINOHOSPITAL.ORG/WOMEN

Suzanne DeSandre, RN, IBCLC

1. Prior to latching the baby		**2. With a Nipple Shield**	
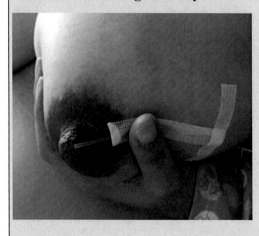	Tape the feeding tube to your breast near the edge of your areola with the end of the on top of your nipple. The tube should extend about ¼ inch past your nipple tip.	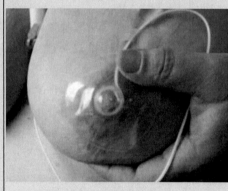	Place feeding tube on top of your nipple and apply nipple shield. The tip of the tube should be in the tip of the shield.

HOW TO FEED BABY WITH A FEEDING TUBE ON YOUR FINGER:

1. **Tape the feeding tube to the pad of a clean index finger** with short finger nail.

2. **Gently introduce your finger with the tube pad side up into the baby's mouth**. Carefully slide your finger along the baby's palate until the baby's lips are close to your first knuckle. Be careful not to gag the baby. The baby should draw your finger in the rest of the way (approximately 1 ½" deep) and start sucking on your finger. Keep your finger straight to help keep the baby's tongue flat & forward.

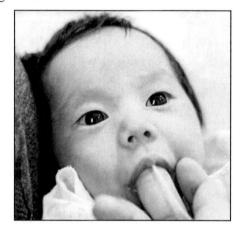

3. **Gently pull down on the baby's chin to roll the lips out**.

4. **Keep bottle no higher than the baby's head and watch for signs of choking or coughing**. Remove finger/tube as needed.

CLEANING THE SNS Starter Kit after each feeding *(from the instruction manual)*:

1. **Fill container halfway with warm soapy water** and force water through tubing, reservoir, and disc/membrane assembly by squeezing reservoir (making sure disc/membrane assembly is inside reservoir lid while cleaning).

2. **Refill with clean water and again** force water through tubing, reservoir and disc/membrane assembly.

3. **Squeeze the empty reservoir a few times** to remove water droplets from the tubing.

4. **Completely disassemble and clean** remaining parts with soapy water. Squeeze reservoir/tubing assembly until the disc/membrane assembly falls out. Use fingernail of forefinger and thumb to remove membrane from disc.

5. **Rinse well and air dry** on a clean towel.

Medela SNS Starter Kits are for sale in the <u>Maternal Connections Gift Store</u>
Open Monday-Friday, 10:00 am – 4:00 pm   *June 2019*

Exclusive Breastfeeding

Exclusive breastfeeding means your baby gets only breast milk without any extra food or drink, not even water.

Tips to help:

- Room-in with your baby in the hospital and room-share at home. Put your baby skin-to-skin as much as possible.

- Let your baby breastfeed often by responding early to your baby's feeding cues.

- *Prolactin* levels are highest at night, so you produce more milk for nighttime feedings.

- Avoid pacifiers and nipples in the first few weeks.

- Giving formula to a breastfeeding baby can have disadvantages. Unless there is a medical reason, there is no need to give formula.

- After feedings, hand express and give any extra milk to your baby.

- Find support through friends, support groups or play groups.

- Contact a lactation consultant if you are having problems breastfeeding.

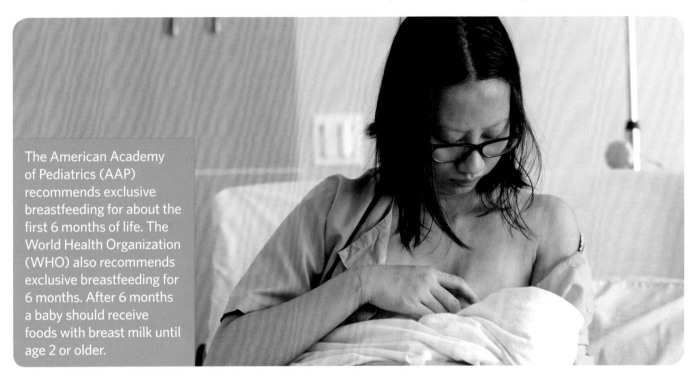

The American Academy of Pediatrics (AAP) recommends exclusive breastfeeding for about the first 6 months of life. The World Health Organization (WHO) also recommends exclusive breastfeeding for 6 months. After 6 months a baby should receive foods with breast milk until age 2 or older.

The Breast

The breasts are delicate organs made of glands, ducts and fatty tissue. The nipple has tiny openings for milk to flow through. These tiny openings are surrounded by muscular tissue that causes the nipple to stand erect when stimulated. Circling the nipple is an area of darker skin called the areola. This area will become darker and larger during pregnancy due to hormonal changes. The areola contains pimple-like structures near its border that are called *Montgomery glands*. These glands secrete an oily substance to lubricate and cleanse the nipple area.

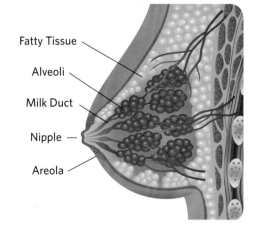

Fatty Tissue

Alveoli

Milk Duct

Nipple —

Areola

Find supporting tools and videos in YoMingo.

Making Milk

Once the placenta is delivered, the level of the hormone progesterone decreases. This sudden drop signals the body to begin making breast milk. To continue making milk, the body needs to keep receiving signals from hormones. When the baby sucks your nipple, this tells your brain to produce two other hormones, prolactin and oxytocin. Prolactin tells your body to make milk. Oxytocin causes the cells around the milk glands to contract and squeeze the milk down the milk ducts and out the nipples. The release of the milk from the milk glands is called the *let-down reflex (or response)*. The let-down reflex may feel like tingling or warmth in the breasts. Some people feel the sensation more than others.

Milk production is regulated by supply and demand. The more milk your baby takes from your breast, the more milk you will make. An emptier breast also makes milk faster than a full one. You will keep your milk production up by breastfeeding your baby as soon as possible after birth and 8 or more times in 24 hours, including at night.

Types of Breast Milk

Colostrum

Colostrum is the first milk you make for your baby. It is easily digested and produced in just the right amount for your baby's small stomach. The more colostrum your baby gets, the more dirty diapers you will see.

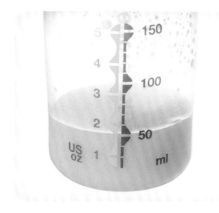

Facts about colostrum:

- Commonly called "Liquid Gold", it can be yellow to clear in color.
- Very high in protein.
- Easily digested.
- Helps prevent low blood sugar.
- Provides protection against infection.
- Coats the stomach and intestines and protects against any invading organisms.

Transitional Milk

Transitional milk occurs as your milk changes character and increases in quantity. When you breastfeed regularly, your breasts will be stimulated to produce transitional milk. The content of this milk includes high levels of fat, lactose and water-soluble vitamins. This milk contains more calories than colostrum and is very high in protein content.

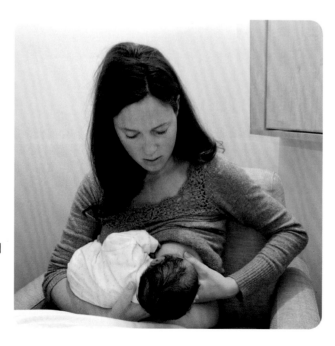

Mature Milk

Your milk will change and increase in amount in about 1 to 3 days. Feeding your baby often in the first few days will help you make the amount of mature milk your baby needs. Mature milk is mostly water, which is necessary to maintain the correct fluid balance for the infant. The rest is comprised of carbohydrates, proteins, and fats that are necessary for both growth and energy. It is also composed of wonderful immunologic properties. These properties do not disappear, but remain throughout breastfeeding.

Breastfeeding Your Baby

Feeding Cues ↺

When your baby is ready to breastfeed they will show feeding cues (signs that they are ready to feed). Keep your baby in the room with you and place your baby skin-to-skin on your chest often. This will help you learn your baby's feeding cues and respond to them quickly.

Your baby may be too upset to breastfeed if they are already crying. In this case, calm your baby first by gently rocking them side to side, or try skin-to-skin contact.

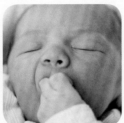

Rooting: Baby's open mouth searching side to side for the breast

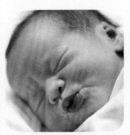

Hands to mouth and stretching

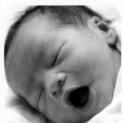

Lip smacking

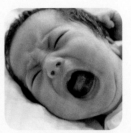

Tongue thrusting and fidgeting

Crying (late cue) and frantic movement

Breastfeeding Positioning

There are several different "holds" you can use when you are breastfeeding. You will likely find one or two that work best for you and your baby. Not all holds work for everyone. No matter which hold you are using, you need to have your baby in the proper position for feeding so they can get enough milk and your nipple will not become sore.

> You will be amazed at how just a slight adjustment in positioning can make a huge difference in comfort for you and your baby.

Guidelines for proper positioning:

- Chest-to-chest.
- Alignment — baby's ear, shoulder and hip in a straight line.
- Support the base of your baby's head.

> Good positioning and latch-on are the keys to successful breastfeeding.

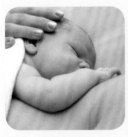

Laid Back

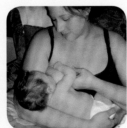

Cradle or "Madonna" Hold

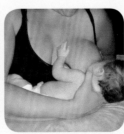

Cross-Cradle or Transitional Hold

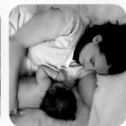

Side-Lying Hold

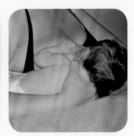

Clutch/Football Hold

↺ Find supporting tools and videos in YoMingo.

Latch-on

When your baby "latches on" to your breast correctly they will have all of the nipple and a good amount of areolar tissue in their mouth. This will give your baby more milk and keep your nipple from becoming sore.

Guidelines for proper latch:

- Before feeding, wash your hands, find a comfortable place and choose a feeding position.
- Skin-to-skin contact can be used before feeding or during a feeding session if your baby isn't ready to latch on.
- Gently massage each breast and hand express until milk comes out. (Follow instructions on page 106)
- Line up your baby's chest with your chest and their nose with your nipple.
- Support your breast and gently lift it. Make sure your fingers are away from the areolar tissue.
- Stroke your baby's upper lip lightly with your nipple in a downward motion, pausing on baby's lower lip, to help their mouth to open wide.
- Be patient until they open their mouth wide. Let them take the lead.
- Your baby's head should be slightly tilted back.
- Aim your nipple toward the roof of their mouth.
- Their chin should come to your breast first.
- When they open wide, quickly and gently pull them toward your breast.
- Their mouth should cover your nipple and more of the lower portion of the areola. This is called an asymmetrical or "off-centered" latch.
- A good latch is a learned response. Be patient with yourself and your baby.

Signs of a good latch:

- All of the nipple and as much of the areola as possible is in baby's mouth.
- Lips are "flanged" or turned out.
- Tongue is over lower gum.
- Baby stays on breast.
- There is no biting or pinching pain.
- Watch for signs of swallowing (long jaw motions).

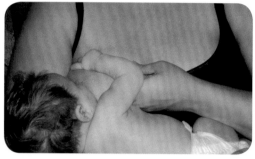

Align baby's nose with your nipple.

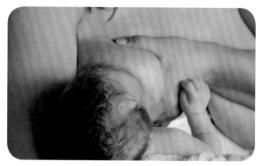

Support breast.

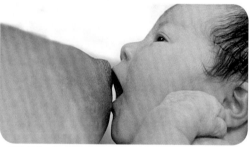

Wait for baby to open their mouth wide. Lower lip is further from nipple.

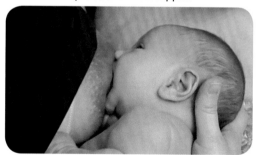

Good positioning makes a good latch possible.

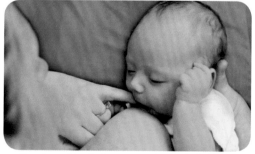

Break suction before removing from breast.

Find supporting tools and videos in YoMingo.

Baby-Led Latch

This leaned-back position, also called biological nursing, is comfortable for both you and your baby. With the baby-led latch position, you are helping your own, and your baby's natural instincts. This position may help your baby to get a better latch and help you relax, too. Make yourself comfortable and lean back with good support for your head, shoulders and arms.

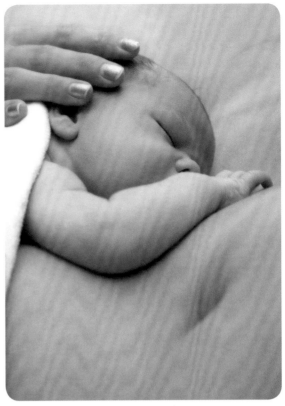

- Let your baby snuggle into your chest. Gravity will help them stay close.

- Place the front of baby's body to the front of your body.

- Let your baby's cheek rest close to your breast. Your baby may start squirming and bobbing their head toward your nipple.

- Support your baby's neck and shoulders with one hand and their hips with the other.

- Follow your baby's lead — when you see their chin hit your breast you may see them open their mouth and latch on.

- Stay calm and relaxed as your baby seeks your breast and allow them to follow their instincts.

Cluster Feeding

Cluster feeding is when your baby feeds close together at certain times of the day. It usually happens in the evening, but all babies are different. Cluster feeding is very common in newborns. Because all of these feedings may work your body overtime, here are some tips to remember:

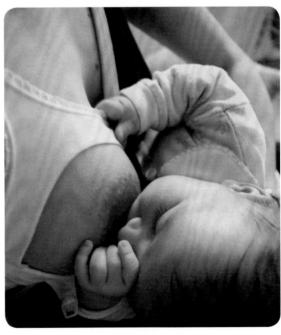

- You are doing nothing wrong — this is normal.

- Make sure you are eating and drinking.

- Make yourself a nest for the day and make sleep a priority.

- Talk to other parents. Get the support you need.

- Ask for help when you need it.

- Let your baby breastfeed whenever they want to.

- Do not supplement your baby with formula. It may decrease your milk supply. Babies who are fed formula still have fussy periods.

- Let your baby instinctively breastfeed and know that the fussy period is just a normal stage in your child's life.

Babies need 8 or more feedings in a 24-hour period.

Is My Baby Eating Enough?

A common concern among new parents is whether their baby is getting enough to eat. The majority of the time they are. It is common to think you do not have enough milk, but, in most cases, you are producing enough. Your baby's stomach is very small at birth and does not need much to fill up. As your baby's stomach grows, they will want to eat more, which stimulates your milk production.

Look for these signs:

- At least 8 feedings in 24 hours.
- Enough wet and dirty diapers for their age.
- Active and alert with a strong cry.
- Mouth and lips are wet and pink.

If you feel your baby is not getting enough milk, contact your healthcare provider or lactation consultant.

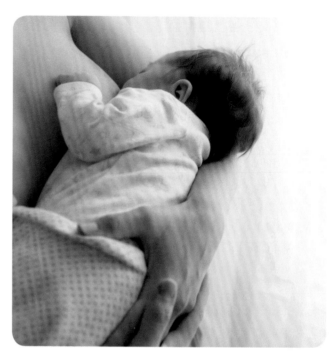

How Big Is Baby's Tummy?

Babies have small tummies, and they need to be fed often so they can grow. It will take a lot of feeding to double their birth weight within 4 to 6 months. Full-term, healthy infants have the ability to regulate their milk intake when they are fed on cue. It is common for babies to feed often during the first few days. This helps bring in a good milk supply.

Approximate Newborn Stomach Size

Day 1
Size of a grape
5 - 7 ml
1 - 1 ½ teaspoon

Day 3
Size of a cherry tomato
22 - 27 ml
1 ½ - 2 tablespoons

Day 7
Size of an apricot
45 - 60 ml
1 ½ - 2 ounces

At 1 month newborn tummies are the size of an egg and hold 80 - 150 ml (3 - 5 ounces).

 Find supporting tools and videos in YoMingo.

Breastfeeding Questions

Will my breasts leak all the time?

This will be different for each person. It's possible for you to have a let-down response when you are not feeding the baby. Applying gentle pressure to the nipple will usually stop the flow of milk. This can be done discreetly by crossing your arms and pressing them against your chest. Disposable or washable breast pads are available to wear on the inside of your bra to protect your clothes from wet spots. Make sure to change them as needed so the dampness does not break down your nipple tissue. Leakage becomes less of a problem as time goes on.

Can I breastfeed if I have had breast surgery?

Several factors can affect your milk production, such as the time since your surgery and the type of surgery. Any type of surgery (biopsy, lumpectomy, lift, reduction, implants) may decrease breast stimulation and interrupt the flow of breast milk. Studies have shown that some women can still be successful with breastfeeding even though they have had these types of breast surgeries. Double pumping may be needed for extra stimulation to the breasts. If needed, a supplemental feeding device can be used to give your baby extra milk while at the breast. Discuss a plan with your lactation consultant. Also review your breast surgery history with your baby's healthcare provider. They will want to carefully monitor your baby's weight gain.

Can I breastfeed if I am taking certain medications?

Many medications pass into the milk, although in very small amounts. Most are not a problem for breastfeeding. There are times when you may need to pump and discard your milk while on a particular medication. Contact your healthcare professional or lactation consultant for the most updated information on a particular medication you are taking.

Is it okay to use alcohol or caffeine while breastfeeding?

As with pregnancy, caffeine and alcohol should be used with caution during lactation. Alcohol is transferred to breast milk. If you choose to have alcohol, it is recommended to wait 2 hours for each drink you had before you begin breastfeeding. Both alcohol and caffeine have been shown to interfere with the breast milk let-down reflex. Caffeine may cause symptoms of colic or irritability in your baby, so avoid it or only have 1 to 2 servings per day.

Do I need to supplement with formula?

Healthy full-term babies do not need supplementation unless it is for medical treatment and breast milk is not available. Formula supplementation for non-medical reasons has some risks. Formula can decrease the healthy bacteria in the baby's intestines that protect against infection. Formula is harder to digest, so baby may not breastfeed as often. This can lead to *engorgement*, a lower milk supply and you not reaching your breastfeeding goals.

Hand Expression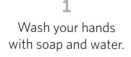

Why is hand expression important?

- Helps reassure you that you have breast milk.
- Helps promote latch and increase milk volume.
- May use to spoon-feed a fussy baby.
- Great companion skill to pumping breast milk.

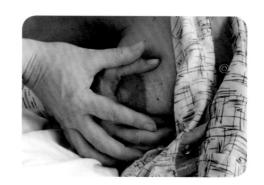

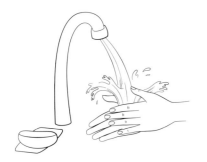 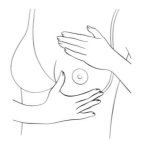 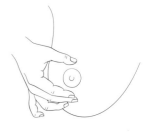

1
Wash your hands with soap and water.

2
Have a clean container, such as a bowl or cup, ready to catch your milk.

3
Gently massage your breasts to make the milk flow more easily. Stroke gently from the top of your breast toward the nipple.

4
Place your hand in a wide, C-shaped hold on the breast.

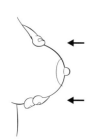 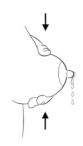

5
Press in toward chest wall.

6
Compress the breast to express milk, then relax. Hand motion should not rub or chafe the skin and fingers shouldn't move on the skin.

7
Rotate your fingers to another position on the breast and repeat.

Find supporting tools and videos in YoMingo.

Human Milk Storage Guidelines

Depending on what study or book you read, these storage tips may vary. Please ask your lactation consultant or healthcare provider for the best storage guidelines and recommendations. If pumping and storing for a premature baby, please talk to your healthcare team about proper storage.

Storage Locations and Temperatures			
TYPE OF BREAST MILK	**COUNTERTOP** 77°F or colder / (25°C) (room temperature)	**REFRIGERATOR** 40°F / (4°C)	**FREEZER** 0°F or colder / (-18°C)
Freshly Expressed or Pumped	Up to **4 hours**	Up to **4 days**	✓ Within **6 months** is best. ✓ Up to **12 months** is acceptable.
Thawed, Previously Frozen	**1-2 hours**	Up to **1 day** (24 hours)	**Never** refreeze human milk after it has been thawed.
Left Over from a Feeding (baby did not finish the bottle)	Use within **2 hours** after the baby is finished feeding.		

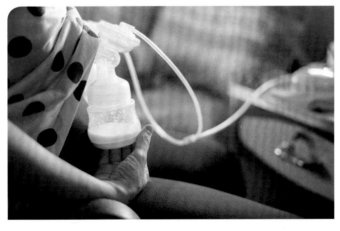

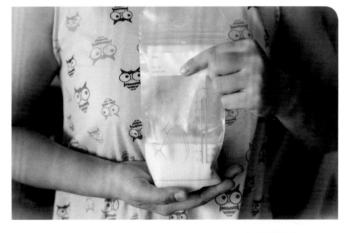

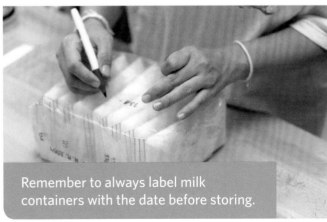

Remember to always label milk containers with the date before storing.

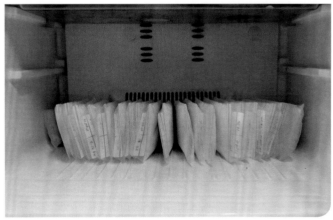

Find supporting tools and videos in YoMingo.

My Baby's Daily Record

		midnight	noon
Day 1:	Goal: at least 8 to 12 nursings	12 1 2 3 4 5 6 7 8 9 10 11	12 1 2 3 4 5 6 7 8 9 10 11
	Wet diaper: W	Black tarry soiled diaper: S	

		midnight	noon
Day 2:	Goal: at least 8 to 12 nursings	12 1 2 3 4 5 6 7 8 9 10 11	12 1 2 3 4 5 6 7 8 9 10 11
	Wet diaper: W W	Brown tarry soiled diaper: S S	

		midnight	noon
Day 3:	Goal: at least 8 to 12 nursings	12 1 2 3 4 5 6 7 8 9 10 11	12 1 2 3 4 5 6 7 8 9 10 11
	Wet diaper: W W W	Green soiled diaper: S S S	

		midnight	noon
Day 4:	Goal: at least 8 to 12 nursings	12 1 2 3 4 5 6 7 8 9 10 11	12 1 2 3 4 5 6 7 8 9 10 11
	Wet diaper: W W W W	Yellow soiled diaper: S S S S	

		midnight	noon
Day 5:	Goal: at least 8 to 12 nursings	12 1 2 3 4 5 6 7 8 9 10 11	12 1 2 3 4 5 6 7 8 9 10 11
	Wet diaper: W W W W W	Yellow soiled diaper: S S S S	

		midnight	noon
Day 6:	Goal: at least 8 to 12 nursings	12 1 2 3 4 5 6 7 8 9 10 11	12 1 2 3 4 5 6 7 8 9 10 11
	Wet diaper: W W W W W W	Yellow soiled diaper: S S S S	

		midnight	noon
Day 7:	Goal: at least 8 to 12 nursings	12 1 2 3 4 5 6 7 8 9 10 11	12 1 2 3 4 5 6 7 8 9 10 11
	Wet diaper: W W W W W W W	Yellow soiled diaper: S S S S	

		midnight	noon
Day 8:	Goal: at least 8 to 12 nursings	12 1 2 3 4 5 6 7 8 9 10 11	12 1 2 3 4 5 6 7 8 9 10 11
	Wet diaper: W W W W W W W	Yellow soiled diaper: S S S S	

		midnight	noon
Day 9:	Goal: at least 8 to 12 nursings	12 1 2 3 4 5 6 7 8 9 10 11	12 1 2 3 4 5 6 7 8 9 10 11
	Wet diaper: W W W W W W W	Yellow soiled diaper: S S S S	

		midnight	noon
Day 10:	Goal: at least 8 to 12 nursings	12 1 2 3 4 5 6 7 8 9 10 11	12 1 2 3 4 5 6 7 8 9 10 11
	Wet diaper: W W W W W W W	Yellow soiled diaper: S S S S	

Please be advised: Some babies may have **more** wet or soiled diapers per day.

If on a certain day your baby has **less** wet diapers and/or less dirty diapers than listed on your breastfeeding log, contact your baby's healthcare provider or lactation consultant.

This log is designed for use with a well, full-term newborn. Ask your baby's healthcare provider what you need to know about breastfeeding your premature or special-needs newborn.

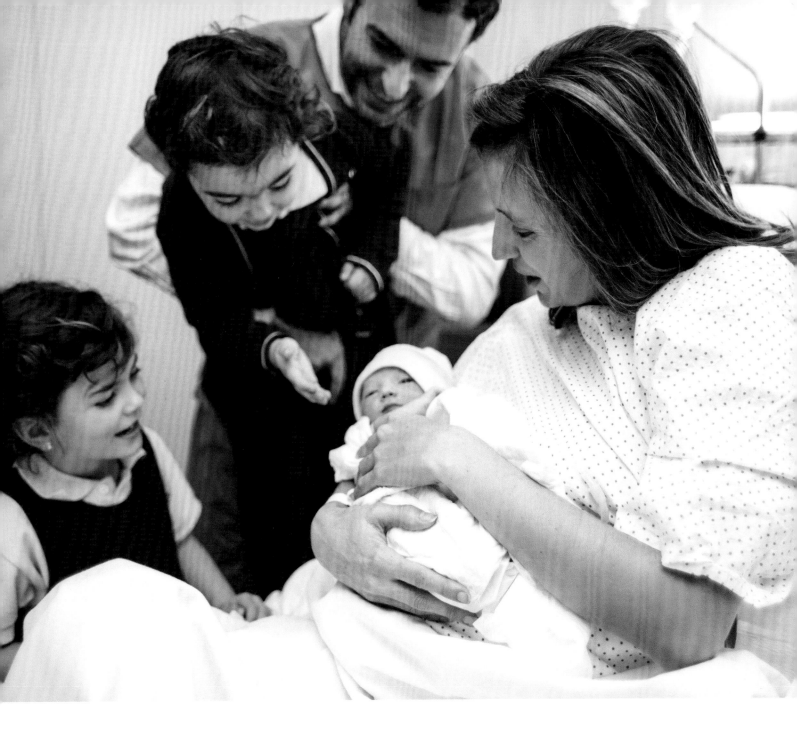

Conclusion

A great deal of how you nurture and love your child comes naturally. Each baby is unique, so honor the individuality of your child as you define your family values. But also know that parenting is a process that requires you to constantly learn. You will discover new skills and insights along the way that will allow you to learn what works best for you, your baby and your family. The success of parenting does not come from the day-to-day responsibilities but instead comes from what you believe and the priorities you set forth. Parenting is possibly the most challenging job you will ever have. You will realize very quickly that parenting is one of the most defining and rewarding responsibilities that outweighs any of life's challenges you may face in the future. Embrace every moment — even the tough times. At the end of the day it comes down to love. Your love for your baby will guide you in making the right decisions. Enjoy your journey!

Contact your healthcare provider for continued support throughout this journey.

Glossary

acrocyanosis: A bluish appearance of the hands and feet of a newborn for the first few hours after birth.

afterbirth cramps: Pain from the uterus contracting after birth to decrease bleeding and return it to prepregnancy size.

amniotic fluid: Water-like fluid that surrounds the baby in the uterus.

amniotic sac (bag of waters): Thin membrane that encloses the developing baby and contains the amniotic fluid. It prevents bacteria from reaching the baby. The bag tears when the "water breaks" and releases the amniotic fluid outside of the body through the vagina.

anesthesia: General or localized pain relief.

apgar test / score: A rating or score given to newborns at 1 and 5 minutes of age. The score is based on 5 categories; color, cry, muscle tone, respiration and reflexes. There is a possible 0 to 2 points for each or a maximum total score of 10.

areola: The dark area around the nipple.

back labor: A condition that occurs in approximately 25% of all labors. The back of the baby's head is directed to the pregnant person's back or turned toward their sacrum, which causes extreme back discomfort.

bilirubin: A yellowish substance formed during the normal breakdown of old red blood cells in the body.

bloody show: Pink or blood-tinged mucous discharge from the vagina that can occur sometime before or during labor.

Braxton Hicks contractions: Intermittent uterine contractions with unpredictable frequency throughout pregnancy. These contractions are most often painless and occur more frequently as pregnancy progresses.

breech: The buttocks or feet of the baby appear first in the birth canal instead of the baby's head.

cesarean birth: The method used to birth a baby through a surgical incision in the abdomen and uterus.

cervix: The neck-like lower part of the uterus that dilates and thins during labor to allow the baby to pass through.

chloasma: The patchy, darkening of the skin or the face due to hormonal changes during pregnancy.

circumcision: The removal of the foreskin of the penis.

coagulation: Clotting of blood.

colostrum: The yellow to almost colorless forerunner to breast milk. It is present in the breasts during pregnancy and is the initial fluid that baby will receive for approximately 3 days until breast milk is established.

contractions: The rhythmical tightening and relaxing of the uterine muscles that cause changes to occur to cervix.

crowning: The appearance of the infant's head at the vaginal opening.

diaphragm: The muscle that separates the chest cavity from the abdominal cavity.

dilation: The gradual opening of the cervix to permit passage of the baby into the vagina. It is measured in centimeters from 0 to 10.

effacement: The gradual thinning, shortening and drawing up of the cervix. This is measured in percentages from 0 to 100%.

electronic fetal monitoring: Using a machine to record baby's heartbeat and uterine contractions. It is placed on the abdomen externally by 2 belts — one applied on the fundus to track contractions and the other placed on the abdomen to pick up the heart rate. Monitoring can be done through the vagina to achieve more accurate readings. An electrode is attached to the baby's scalp to monitor baby's heart rate, and a pressure catheter is inserted through the cervix into the uterus to measure strength of contractions.

enema: A tube is placed into the rectum and fluid is inserted to start a bowel movement.

engorgement: Swelling of the breasts after giving birth caused by milk, blood flow and other fluids. This can cause the breasts to feel hard and painful.

episiotomy: A surgical incision of the perineum that enlarges the vaginal opening for birth of the baby.

epidural anesthesia: Regional anesthesia administered through the patient's back by a thin flexible tube placed in the epidural space. It numbs the lower part of the body.

fontanelles (soft spots): Gaps between the bones in the baby's head that allow for shaping through the birth canal during the birth process.

forceps: Instruments used while pushing to assist the baby in moving under the pubic bone or through the lower part of the birth canal.

fundus: The rounded upper portion of the uterus (womb).

genital herpes: A virus that is characterized by small sores in clusters on the genitals. The infection is generally sexually transmitted and can affect the baby.

gestation: The period of time a baby is carried in the uterus. It is usually described in weeks, with 40 weeks being full term.

Group Beta Strep: A bacterial infection that can be found in the pregnant persons vagina or rectum and can be passed to the baby during birth.

hemorrhoid: A dilated blood vessel inside the anus and beneath its thin lining (internal) or outside the anus and beneath the surface of the skin (external).

hormone: A chemical substance produced in the body that is carried through the blood stream and causes the function of another gland.

induction: The use of medications or amniotomy (rupture of membranes) to stimulate labor contractions.

insomnia: The inability to sleep.

jaundice: A newborn condition caused by excess yellow bilirubin pigment. Treatment may be required but it is generally not necessary.

Kegel exercises: An exercise contracting the pelvic floor muscles that improves pelvic floor muscle tone and helps prevent urinary incontinence.

lanugo: Fine hair that covers the baby's body and may be seen at birth.

let-down reflex or response (milk ejection reflex): The release of milk from the milk glands stimulated by the baby during nursing.

lightening: The sensation of the baby "dropping" as the baby descends into the pelvic cavity.

linea nigra: A line running from the navel to the pubic hair line that darkens during pregnancy because of hormonal changes.

Glossary

local anesthesia: The numbing of a certain area with anesthetic medication.

lochia: The discharge from the uterus during the 6-week period following birth (postpartum).

meconium: The greenish black material that collects in the baby's intestines as they develop in the uterus. It will become the first bowel movement the baby has.

meditation: Focusing your mind on a thought, object or activity to help you relax and create calmness.

milia: White spots on the baby's nose and cheeks that disappear over time.

meconium: A greenish material that collects in the bowels of a developing baby that is normally expelled after birth. It can stain amniotic fluid if expelled before birth.

molding: The shaping of the baby's head during labor to adjust to the size and shape of the birth canal.

Mongolian spots: A bluish pigmented area on the shoulders or near the base of the spine that is present at birth and usually disappears during childhood.

Montgomery glands: Pimple-like structures on the areola. These glands secrete a substance that aids in lubricating and cleansing the area.

mucous plug: A thick mucous plug that develops in the cervix early in pregnancy due to hormone shifts. It protects the pregnant uterus from bacteria present in the vagina.

multipara: A person who has given birth to more than one child.

oxytocin: A hormone in the body that contributes to the start of labor and later stimulates the "let-down" response for breastfeeding.

patient-controlled analgesia: Pain relieving medications delivered through an IV pump.

pelvis: The basin-shaped ring of bones at the bottom of the body that connects the spinal column to the legs. It is composed of two hip bones (iliac) that join in the front (pubic bones) and back (sacrum).

perineal: Relating to the perineum.

perineum: The layers of muscles and tissues between the vagina and rectum.

phototherapy: Treatment of jaundice in a newborn through light therapy.

pitocin: A synthetic oxytocin used to induce or enhance labor. Also given after delivery of the placenta to contract the uterus.

placenta: The circular, flat organ in the pregnant uterus that serves as the exchange station for nutrients and oxygen. It is delivered after the baby and is often referred to as the "afterbirth."

postpartum depression and anxiety disorders: Conditions that can occur in up to 10% of people who recently gave birth. It most likely results from changing physiology, certain hormones and other changes such as self-image, lifestyle, stress and fatigue. It is a treatable condition.

postpartum: The 6-week period of time after the birth of a baby.

premature infant (preterm): An infant born before 37 weeks gestation.

presentation: Refers to the part of the baby that is lying closest to the cervix.

primipara: A person having their first child.

prolactin: A hormone secreted from the pituitary gland that stimulates the milk gland cells in the breast to begin producing milk.

prostaglandin: A chemical substance that causes uterine contractions.

restitution: The return of the rotated head of the baby to its natural alignment with the shoulders.

rooting: The tendency of an infant to open their mouth and turn toward an object. It can be elicited by gently stroking their cheek or corner of their mouth.

round ligament pain: Pain in one or both groin regions from stretching or spasm of the round ligaments.

station: Indicates the location of the baby's head in the pelvis in relation to the bony ischial spines of the pelvis.

stork bite: a playful name for a birthmark.

stretch marks: Silver or red streaks or stripes on the skin, especially on the abdomen. Caused by the stretching of the skin during pregnancy.

transitional milk: Colostrum is replaced by a creamy white milk called transitional milk before the mature breast milk is established.

transverse lie: A horizontal (sideways) position of the baby in the uterus.

trimester: A period of 3 months. One-third of a full-term pregnancy.

umbilical cord: Structure that contains blood vessels that connect the baby to the placenta. The cord contains one vein to transport nourishment to the baby and two arteries to remove wastes from baby.

urinary catheter: A flexible tube that is placed through the urethra into the bladder to drain it of retained urine.

uterus: The muscular organ that contains the products of conception — the baby, placenta, membranes, amniotic fluid and umbilical cord. It contracts during labor to move the baby through the birth canal. It is commonly referred to as the womb.

vacuum extractor: A special instrument that is attached to the baby's head to help guide them out of the birth canal.

vagina: The lower part of the birth canal that is normally 5 to 6 inches long.

VBAC: "Vaginal Birth After Cesarean"

vernix: A greasy, white material that coats the baby at birth.

Bibliography

AAP Recommended Immunization Schedules. American Academy of Pediatrics Web Site. December 2017 www.aap.org/immunization/izschedule.html.

AAP Updates Recommendation on Car Seats. American Academy of Pediatrics Web Site. Web. 21 Mar. 2011. https://www.aap.org/en-us/about-the-aap/aap-press-room/Pages/AAP-Updates-Recommendation-on-Car-Seats.aspx.

About Sudden Unexpected Infant Death and Sudden Infant Death Syndrome. Centers for Disease Control and Prevention. Centers for Disease Control and Prevention, 29 Sept. 2014. Web. 19 Oct. 2014.

Academy of Breastfeeding Medicine Protocol Committee. (2009). ABM clinical protocol# 3: hospital guidelines for the use of supplementary feedings in the healthy term breastfed neonate, revised 2009. Breastfeeding Medicine, 4(3), 175-182.

American Academy of Pediatrics. (2011). AAP expands guidelines for infant sleep safety and SIDS risk reduction. American Academy of Pediatrics press release.

American Academy of Pediatrics. (2017). AAP reaffirms breastfeeding guidelines. 2012.

American College of Obstetricians and Gynecologists. (1997). Planning for Pregnancy, Birth, and Beyond. Amer College of Obstetricians &.

American College of Obstetricians and Gynecologists. (2006). ACOG Practice Bulletin. Clinical Management Guidelines for Obstetrician-Gynecologists, Number 71, April 2006. Episiotomy. Obstetrics and gynecology, 107(4), 957-62.

American College of Obstetricians and Gynecologists. (2010). ACOG Practice bulletin no. 115: Vaginal birth after previous cesarean delivery. Obstetrics and gynecology, 116(2 Pt 1), 450.

Amir, L. H., & Academy of Breastfeeding Medicine Protocol Committee. (2014). ABM clinical protocol# 4: Mastitis, revised March 2014. Breastfeeding Medicine, 9(5), 239-243.

Boies, E. G., Vaucher, Y. E., & Academy of Breastfeeding Medicine. (2016). ABM Clinical Protocol# 10: Breastfeeding the late preterm (34-36 6/7 weeks of gestation) and early term infants (37-38 6/7 weeks of gestation), second revision 2016. Breastfeeding Medicine, 11(10), 494-500.

Brancato, R. M., Church, S., & Stone, P. W. (2008). A meta-analysis of passive descent versus immediate pushing in nulliparous women with epidural analgesia in the second stage of labor. Journal of Obstetric, Gynecologic & Neonatal Nursing, 37(1), 4-12.

Briere, C. E., Lucas, R., McGrath, J. M., Lussier, M., & Brownell, E. (2015). Establishing breastfeeding with the late preterm infant in the NICU. Journal of Obstetric, Gynecologic, & Neonatal Nursing, 44(1), 102-113.

Britton, C., McCormick, F. M., Renfrew, M. J., Wade, A., & King, S. E. (2007). Support for breastfeeding mothers. Cochrane database of systematic reviews, (1).

Byington, C. L., Maldonado, Y. A., Barnett, E. D., Campbell, J. D., Davies, H. D., Lynfield, R., ... & Rathore, M. H. (2017). Recommended childhood and adolescent immunization schedule-United States, 2017. Pediatrics, 139(3).

Car Seats Recommendations for Children | National Highway Traffic Safety Administration (NHTSA). Home | National Highway Traffic Safety Administration (NHTSA). Web. 2 Jan. 2019. https://www.nhtsa.gov/sites/nhtsa.dot.gov/files/documents/carseatrecommendationsforchildren.pdf

Caring for Your Baby and Young Child: Birth to Age 5 (© 2009 American Academy of Pediatrics) https://www.healthychildren.org/English/ages-stages/baby/bathing-skin-care/Pages/Umbilical-Cord-Care.aspx Last Updated 5/12/2011.

CDC. Are special precautions required for handling breast milk? 2015. Available at https://www.cdc.gov/breastfeeding/ faq/#Precautions (accessed June 26, 2017).

CDC. Proper Storage and Preparation of Breast Milk. May 14, 2018. Available at https://www.cdc.gov/breastfeeding/recommendations/handling_breastmilk.htm (accessed May 31, 2018)

Choose My Plate. Jan 26, 2018 available at https://www.choosemyplate.gov/

Christensson, K., Siles, C., Moreno, L., Belaustequi, A., De La Fuente, P., Lagercrantz, H., ... & Winberg, J. (1992). Temperature, metabolic adaptation and crying in healthy full-term newborns cared for skin-to-skin or in a cot. Acta paediatrica, 81(6-7), 488-493.

Christian, C. W., & Block, R. (2009). Abusive head trauma in infants and children. Pediatrics, 123(5), 1409-1411.

Colson, S. D., Meek, J. H., & Hawdon, J. M. (2008). Optimal positions for the release of primitive neonatal reflexes stimulating breastfeeding. Early Human Development, 84(7), 441-449.

Dekker, R. (2014). Friedman's curve and failure to progress: A leading case of unplanned C-sections.

Dewey, K. G., Cohen, R. J., Brown, K. H., & Rivera, L. L. (2001). Effects of exclusive breastfeeding for four versus six months on maternal nutritional status and infant motor development: results of two randomized trials in Honduras. The Journal of nutrition, 131(2), 262-267.

Dyson, L., McCormick, F., & Renfrew, M. J. (2005). Interventions for promoting the initiation of breastfeeding.(Cochrane Review). In the Cochrane Library (Issue 4).

Eglash, A., & Simon, L. (2017). ABM Clinical Protocol# 8: Human Milk Storage Information for Home Use for Full-Term Infants, Revised 2017. Breastfeeding Medicine, 12(7), 390-395.

Eidelman, A. I., Schanler, R. J., Johnston, M., Landers, S., Noble, L., Szucs, K., & Viehmann, L. (2012). Breastfeeding and the use of human milk. Pediatrics, 129(3), e827-e841.

Ferber, S. G., & Makhoul, I. R. (2004). The effect of skin-to-skin contact (kangaroo care) shortly after birth on the neurobehavioral responses of the term newborn: a randomized, controlled trial. Pediatrics, 113(4), 858-865.

Fleischman, A. R., Oinuma, M., & Clark, S. L. (2010). Rethinking the definition of "term pregnancy". Obstetrics & Gynecology, 116(1), 136-139.

Friedman, A. M., Ananth, C. V., Prendergast, E., D'alton, M. E., & Wright, J. D. (2015). Variation in and factors associated with use of episiotomy. Jama, 313(2), 197-199.

Frisch, M., Aigrain, Y., Barauskas, V., Bjarnason, R., Boddy, S. A., Czauderna, P., ... & Gahr, M. (2013). Cultural bias in the AAP's 2012 Technical Report and Policy Statement on male circumcision. Pediatrics, peds-2012.

Hale, T. W. (2017). Hale & Hartmann's Textbook of Human Lactation. Springer Publishing Company Incorporated.

Hale, T. W., & Rowe, H. E. (2016). Medications and Mothers' Milk 2017. Springer Publishing Company.

Hauck, F. R., Thompson, J. M., Tanabe, K. O., Moon, R. Y., & Vennemann, M. M. (2011). Breastfeeding and reduced risk of sudden infant death syndrome: a meta-analysis. Pediatrics, 128(1), 103-110.

How to Clean, Sanitize, and Store Infant Feeding Items. April 11, 2017. Available at https://www.cdc.gov/healthywater/hygiene/healthychildcare/infantfeeding/cleansanitize.html

Jones, F., & Tully, M. R. (2011). Best practice for expressing, storing and handling human milk: In hospitals, homes and child care settings. Human milk banking association of North America.

Karp, H. N. (2008). Safe swaddling and healthy hips: don't toss the baby out with the bathwater. Pediatrics, 121(5), 1075-1076.

Keefe, M. R. (1987). Comparison of neonatal nighttime sleep-wake patterns in nursery versus rooming-in environments. Nursing research.

Kellams, A., Harrel, C., Omage, S., Gregory, C., Rosen-Carole, C., & Academy of Breastfeeding Medicine. (2017). ABM clinical protocol# 3: Supplementary feedings in the healthy term breastfed neonate, revised 2017. Breastfeeding Medicine, 12(4), 188-198.

Kerkhoff Gromada, K. (2006). Breastfeeding Multiples. New Beginnings, 23(6), pp. 244-249. Retrieved December 28, 2012 from llli.org/nb/nbnovdec06p244.html.

Kim, P., & Swain, J. E. (2007). Sad dads: paternal postpartum depression. Psychiatry (edgmont), 4(2), 35.

Lai, Y. L., Hung, C. H., Stocker, J., Chan, T. F., & Liu, Y. (2015). Postpartum fatigue, baby-care activities, and maternal-infant attachment of vaginal and cesarean births following rooming-in. Applied Nursing Research, 28(2), 116-120.

Lawrence, R. A., & Lawrence, R. M. (2010). Breastfeeding E-Book: A Guide for the Medical Professional. Elsevier Health Sciences.

Medoff-Cooper, B., Bakewell-Sachs, S., Buus-Frank, M. E., & Santa-Donato, A. (2005). The AWHONN Near-Term Infant Initiative: a conceptual framework for optimizing health for near-term infants. Journal of Obstetric, Gynecologic & Neonatal Nursing, 34(6), 666-671.

Mohrbacher, N. (2010). Breastfeeding answers made simple: A guide for helping mothers (pp. 795-798). Amarillo, TX: Hale Publishing.

Mohrbacher, N. (2014). Working and breastfeeding made simple. Praeclarus Press, LLC.

Montgomery, A., & Hale, and The Academy of Breastfeeding Medicine, T. W. (2012). ABM clinical protocol# 15: analgesia and anesthesia for the breastfeeding mother, revised 2012. Breastfeeding Medicine, 7(6), 547-553.

Moore, E. R., Bergman, N., Anderson, G. C., & Medley, N. (2016). Early skin-to-skin contact for mothers and their healthy newborn infants. The Cochrane Library

National Institutes of Health. National Institute of Child Health and Human Development. SIDS: Back to Sleep Campaign.

New Evidence Points to Greater Benefits of Infant Circumcision, But Final Say Is Still Up to Parents, Says AAP. N.p., n.d. Web. 27 Jan. 2015.

Newman, J., & Pitman, T. (2006). The Ultimate Breastfeeding Book of Answers: The Most Comprehensive Problem-solving Guide to Breastfeeding from the Foremost Expert in North America. Harmony.

Nichols, F. H., & Humenick, S. S. (2000). Childbirth education: practice, research and theory. WB Saunders Company.

Pound, C. M., & Unger, S. L. (2012). The baby-friendly initiative: protecting, promoting and supporting breastfeeding. Paediatrics & child health, 17(6), 317-321.

Price, C. T., & Schwend, R. M. (2011). Improper swaddling a risk factor for developmental dysplasia of hip. American Academy of Pediatrics News, 32(11).

Reece-Stremtan, S., Marinelli, K. A., & Academy of Breastfeeding Medicine. (2015). ABM clinical protocol# 21: guidelines for breastfeeding and substance use or substance use disorder, revised 2015. Breastfeeding Medicine, 10(3), 135-141.

Schwarz, E. B., Ray, R. M., Stuebe, A. M., Allison, M. A., Ness, R. B., Freiberg, M. S., & Cauley, J. A. (2009). Duration of lactation and risk factors for maternal cardiovascular disease. Obstetrics and gynecology, 113(5), 974.

Task Force on Sudden Infant Death Syndrome. (2011). SIDS and other sleep-related infant deaths: expansion of recommendations for a safe infant sleeping environment. Pediatrics, peds-2011.

Tohotoa, J., Maycock, B., Hauck, Y. L., Howat, P., Burns, S., & Binns, C. W. (2009). Dads make a difference: an exploratory study of paternal support for breastfeeding in Perth, Western Australia. International breastfeeding journal, 4(1), 15.

Your pregnancy and childbirth: month to month. (2016). Washington, DC: American College of Obstetricians and Gynecologists Washington, DC

Wambach, K., & Riordan, J. (Eds.). (2014). Breastfeeding and human lactation. Jones & Bartlett Learning.